What If It All Goes Right?

Practicing Hope in the Hardest Times

Scarlet Keys

This book is dedicated to
anyone facing the hardest thing.

ISBN: 979-8-218-33988-3

"Crepe Skin"
© 2022 by Little Jay Bird Music/ASCAP
All Rights Reserved

© 2024 by Hoppas Books
All Rights Reserved

Contents

Acknowledgments iv
Preface v
1. Hope 1
2. Everything I've Got 4
3. Boundaries 10
4. Nap Brag: A Call to Inaction 15
5. What Would Henry Do? 19
6. Being Your Own Bodyguard 23
7. The Sound of Quiet 28
8. The "S" Word 30
9. Antidotes to Stress 32
10. Joy 38
11. The Self-Love Club 42
12. Nature 46
13. Hard Gifts 49
14. Good Vibes Only 52
15. Words Matter 58
16. The "F" Word 63
17. Altars in the Day 67
18. Good Morning, Beautiful 71
19. The Alchemy of Gratitude 74
20. Laughter 81
21. Friendship 88
22. A Good Cry .... 93 ✓
23. What's Your Soundtrack? 98
24. Awe and Wonder 106
25. Woo-Woo 113
26. What If It All Goes Right? 116
27. New Management 122
28. Fragile Faith 129
29. Finding Fun 132
30. Tigger and Eeyore 138
31. The Hardest Thing 143
Afterword 151

Acknowledgments

I would like to thank my husband Greg; my daughter Claire; my editor Jonathan Feist; artist Rachel Kice for her heart painting; Monica Dorley for graphic design; Shawn Girsberger for production consulting; Mim Adkins for the author photo; Dr. Molly Buzdon; Hilary Crowley, Ben Glover; Dr. Peter Georges; Jeri, Patte, Tammy, Mary, Jenny, Sarah, Matthew, Luke, Dan, Marcy, Stephanie, Kristin, Michelle, Paul, Shelly, Carina, Susan, Dino, Jamie, Kris, Kathy, Karen, Becca, Tim, Pratt, Marci, Jesse, Liz, Ellen, Claire, Chrissy, Angel, Danielle, Jennifer, Anna, Sally, Jenny, Carolanne, Kate, Rene, Getit, Liz, Joie, Pat, Rebecca, Jack, Pearl, Adam, Jesse, Johnny, Susan, Alyson, Glenda, Carolyn, Rob, Peggy, Rene, Erin, Roger, Rodney; my Berklee family; my amazing students; the Wild Valentine café; and everyone whose kindness and love played a part in my healing and in the making of this book.

Preface

Cancer was a word that I never thought would belong to me, until it did. Once you hear your own name in the same sentence with the "C" word, you are never the same. Hopefully, you eventually become better.

This was the hardest thing that I have ever had to face, but somehow, I realized that I could choose how I was going to go through it. If I had to go through hell, then I would pack well for the trip. I wasn't going to travel lightly. I packed everything: hope, gratitude, joy, laughter, loved ones, faith, trust, and of course, music. I mean, if you're going to walk through hell, who says you can't dance through the flames?

The result was this book. It is about the bravery of hope and the silver linings that come from the rubble of our hardest thing.

During the past two years, I have been on a quest to live better, wider, and more deeply. There are so many unexpected gifts that have come from this difficult time, such as discovering my own bravery and learning to keep my heart more open. I hope that by sharing my experiences and lessons learned, it will help you also reflect on how you are living and perhaps make adjustments that will lead you to live more deliberately.

Scarlet Keys

This book doesn't go into the details of treatment. Other sources discuss what that entails. Rather, it is meant to provide inspiration. Open it to any chapter that you are drawn to, on any given day. Each chapter is only a couple of pages long. Even if you are tired, you can still find something to uplift you.

I hope it will sit by your bedside table and that you will give it to a friend. Most of all, I hope it will provide welcome companionship and support, as you go through your own hardest thing.

1. Hope

"Hope" is the thing with feathers –
That perches in the soul –
And sings the tune without words –
And never stops – at all –

—Emily Dickinson

During the past few years, while I was facing my hardest thing, hope was riding shotgun.

Hope has always come naturally for me. Before my diagnosis, if you had asked me if I was a hopeful person, I would have said yes, of course I am. The truth is, I had never really had my hope challenged or been called to examine my relationship with this optimistic word. But life is not always sunlit. It can be dark, with only a faint glow of light to work in.

Sometimes, though, a glint is all we need.

Lately, hope feels like the most important word in the world. A glint I have needed to get through my hardest thing. It is both fragile and bold.

Hope is a daily and sometimes moment-to-moment practice. Life is better with hope, like sunshine on a cloudy day.

Now, hope is no longer a given or something I just keep folded in my back pocket. These days, I deliberately unfold hope in broad daylight, at midnight, in hospital waiting rooms, and while waiting for test results or anticipating upcoming procedures.

Hope is easy when it's attached to little things, like "I hope to see you at the party" or "I hope we make it to the airport." It asks so much more of us in moments like, "I hope my dad makes it through his surgery" or "I hope my doctor says I'm in remission."

Radical hope is sometimes what we need the most—fierce and active, made of willpower and grit. Bursting with possibility in the direction of the best possible outcome.

Sure, hope can feel like a glittery concept that belongs to Pollyanna or Hallmark cards, in the same trite/cliché category as "Cheer up!" or "Hold on!" It can feel distant as the moon—far out of reach.

But being hopeful is a little bit badass. It is brave and beautiful to be hopeful.

Just reading the word "hope" makes us feel better. But beyond its mere existence, hope needs to be busy doing things and making plans to make the situation better or to reach a goal. Hope shares the same air as Optimism, but it is more grounded in reality.

When Hope is asked to attend to more difficult things, we might have to invite Trust and Faith along to help. Hope is stronger when it walks arm-in-arm with Faith and Trust. They hold the energy of great expectations. Together, they roll up their sleeves and do what needs to be done.

Sometimes, we have to practice hope. When we can hold it, hope gets us through our hardest times. We can achieve an elevated state of being and come to embody it. There is a brilliant expectant energy to it, like a firework waiting to be lit.

Being hopeful measurably improves our mental health, combats depression and loneliness, and can even lower our risk of cancer and other health issues, according to psychologist Charles Snyder. Being hopeful is crucial to thriving.

When we practice hope, it eventually defines who we are and how we look at the world. We then become the people who look for the best, aim for the best, and work toward the desired outcome.

What would this world be without hope? Hope makes us get out of bed in the morning. It makes us try again. It inspires the scientist to find a cure and the heart to love again. Hope was the one thing that allowed me to let in joy and gratitude and even laughter and fun. Hope is the light that stands guard against the darkness so that we can let go and sink into the loveliest emotions that put our hearts at ease.

Hope isn't a guarantee that things will go well. It's just a very confident hunch that they just might, and that is the feeling that has saved me.

In Practice

- What are some ways you can practice hope?
- How can you infuse this moment and this day, with an expectation for the highest outcome?
- What can you do to take action towards achieving the best outcome?

2. Everything I've Got

*"There are four questions of value in life....
What is sacred? Of what is the spirit made?
What is worth living for, and what is worth
dying for? The answer to each is the same.
Only love."*

—Lord Byron

I had a friend who had been diagnosed with advanced cancer, and he didn't want to tell anyone. He didn't want to face his friends with their tilted heads or hear the concern lining their voices, and wanted to avoid the sympathy and the fuss. I encouraged him to share what he was going through, because people who love us *want* to *love* us. They want to be a part of our journey and our healing in any way they can. It's a gift to let the people who care about us care for us.

I am someone who needs a get-well card and a meal train for a hangnail, so when I received a serious health diagnosis, I needed to tell everyone I knew what was going on, because I knew it was going to take everything to get me through it.

The weird part is that, sometimes, the people you thought were going to show up for you, don't or can't,

What If It All Goes Right?

for some reason, and the people you barely know or never thought would be there show up.

It isn't always easy, but we have to find a way to offer grace to the people who let us down or don't meet our expectations. They might not know how to cope with what we are going through or don't know how to be close to illness or trauma.

I broke the news via texts, phone calls, and public posts on Facebook.

My friend and one of my favorite songwriters texted, "How are you?" I texted back "It's going to take everything I have to get me through," and he said "Well, it's a good thing you've got everything." I loved that, and of course, being a songwriter, I wrote it down.

I was stunned at the outpouring of love and support that came from the most unexpected places. Dinners were set up and delivered on my back porch by a group of local moms. A friend of mine set me up with a monthly delivery of insanely expensive probiotic yogurt made from coconut milk. My next-door neighbor tracked down a nursery that sold her favorite rose bush and planted it outside her house, positioned so that I look out my living room window and see something beautiful.

My lifetime friend from Sweden flew over and took me directly to a Lizzo concert. She bought sets of books and sent me one while she read the other so we could read them at the same time, and said, "You can go to the edge of the water's wave and touch the ocean in New Hampshire, and I will reach into the cold North Sea at the same time so we can say hello."

Past students sent me cards, cozy blankets, journals, Alicia Keys' organic skin products "from one Keys to the other." Another friend gave me free zoom hypnotherapy sessions.

One of my favorite local artists dropped off a small gold and red painting that had one word written off to the side that just said "Shit." That painting has now been passed from woman to woman going through breast cancer. We call it the traveling shit painting.

I was amazed at how other woman who had gone through cancer were willing to meet with me. I had a Zoom session with a woman who shared her journey and talked about radiation, and then asked, "Do you want to see my boobs?" She generously pulled up her shirt and shared her scars and her heart.

I met a woman at a music show who had gone through a mastectomy and reconstruction who offered to show me the results in the bathroom because she was thrilled. I was so grateful for the offer, because finding pictures of reconstruction online can be scary. We went into the bathroom, she took off her shirt, and then reached back to undo her bra and stopped and said "Wait, what's your name again?" and I said "I'll tell you after, it will be funnier that way."

An old friend of mine had gone through breast cancer, and although we hadn't spoken in years, she would FaceTime me at treatment, take late night calls and keep saying, "Before you know it, you will be through this."

What If It All Goes Right?

My husband was endlessly supportive with foot rubs and dancing on command to ABBA or a raunchy rap song just to make me laugh at midnight. After my surgery, he said, "Oh honey, I'm a leg man, and now when we hug, you are so much closer." I tucked those lies into my heart, and am so grateful for him.

Love is real. It's made of something that can hold you when you can't hold yourself, like a huge airplane riding rippled air. Knowing we are loved, knowing we are thought about, is everything.

It was awkward and hard being on the receiving end, but it is beautifully awkward and life-affirming.

My sister was on dialysis for years. She once said, "Never ask someone what they need, just *show up* with it."

When people said, "Let me know what you need, don't hesitate to ask," I was totally uncomfortable with asking for help or dinner or anything. What was I going to ask for? "Oh, can you bring me a tuna fish sandwich and tap dance on my doorstep?" Or "Can you drive by my house real slow, playing 'Thriller' out your car window," or "Parachute into my yard with a thousand daisies?" No, what I've learned is you just bring the dinner, you send the flowers, you just show up, because people are too uncomfortable to ask.

Over the time of treatment, I was amazed at how I was held by love. There were so many days I'd be out in my yard crying as I was coming down off the steroids, and then I'd get a card in the mail or a care package so thoughtfully picked and their love literally lifted me up. Love was a palpable thing. Knowing that we matter is a balm to the soul.

I got a handwritten letter in the mail from a past student that said, "I know this paper must feel strange, but that's because it has seeds in it. Turn this paper over, and write down what you want to see grow, and then plant it in the ground." Another student sent me a huge soft purple blanket and a journal and a care package with CBD lip gloss and a Wonder Woman doll.

It all got me through.

I had friends play piano for me on Zoom, send me funny videos, my friend and his wife brought me an orchid and read me poems, my work friends sent gift cards and there were so many wonderful gestures that made a bad day better.

I say all of this because I think these creative and thoughtful things are wonderful ideas to offer to friends and family when they go through their hardest thing.

A care package can change the day. For the person struggling and facing down uncertainty, getting a box delivered means more than we might imagine. When someone takes the time to put a care package together, it's such an unexpected surprise. You open the box, sift through the tissue paper, the pretty wrapping, the handwritten card, the little things someone picked out for you, and mostly, the thought that went into putting it together and sending it, and you are lifted up by their thoughtfulness.

What If It All Goes Right?

I eventually wrote that song idea I stole from a songwriter friend, and one of the lines is "It's gonna take everything I've got, so it's a good thing that I've got everything."

No matter what we are going through, we need our friends. We need everything.

> ### In Practice
> - Let your friends and loved ones know what's going on with you.
> - Ask at least two people for help.
> - See if you can ask a good friend to ask others for help on your behalf.
> - When you're having a hard day, see what you can do to help someone else by sending a text, sending a card or flowers, etc.

3. Boundaries

"Good fences make good neighbors."

—Robert Frost

I'd always imagined what my reaction would be to facing something life-threatening. I thought there would be a lot of seizing the day and bucket-list additions. I would leap out of bed each morning like I'd been shot out of a canon, and there would suddenly be a lot of skipping for some reason, and I'd be throwing glitter at the day. Maybe learn to scuba dive and fly to Machu Picchu, and never be irritated ever again.

But what came up instead was the question of what needed to be changed in my life, and how I really wanted to spend my time. It turns out that I needed to learn how to set and hold boundaries.

How was a people-pleasing codependent supposed to build fences around her time and energy? My parents came from the south, so I have the southern hostess heritage, and I am a woman still shaking off the gender role expectations of volunteering, cleaning, cooking, shopping, all correspondence (thank you cards, birthday reminders), entertaining guests, and making polite conversation.

What If It All Goes Right?

After going from the fast lane to the breakdown lane, my life was begging for the middle lane. But I was also a workaholic and a mom, so words like "moderation" and "ease" felt like a shirt that was too tight. I wasn't blaming myself for getting sick, but I was retracing my steps and examining the way I'd been living.

The dreaded and complicated word "boundary" felt rude, like I was putting up electric fences with barbed wire around myself and my time.

How dare I say no or not carry all the conversation at family gatherings or go lie down in the middle of a party when I am tired?

Saying no and setting boundaries felt like I was letting people down. But when you are going through a challenging time, like a death in the family, divorce, the loss of a job, or chemo, you have a built-in boundary: you actually *can't* talk on the phone or make small talk or handle someone else's adult drama because you are busy wrestling grief, loss, or a job change, or tasked with saving your own life.

The word "no" is the quickest route to setting a boundary.

So I started small, practicing with, "I'm so sorry, I wish I could, but I just can't." Moving on to "No thank you," and graduating to "no."

Tone of voice can really help with the way the "no" lands. You can say it in the warm velvety voice of a meditation teacher, and it comes off more as a gift than a rejection.

I heard about someone who was starting to get famous. The demands on their time were becoming difficult to accommodate, so they started saying, "That's just not possible." If we are wishy-washy and our boundary seems porous, people might push a little. So I really like "I'm sorry, it's just not possible." It's really hard to argue with.

It's important to practice saying no and not chasing after it like you dropped a stack of papers, scrambling to pick them all up while apologizing profusely. Just say one of the shortest words in the English language, "No," and then let the silence that follows hang in the air unattended to.

We need boundaries around our time, our schedule, and more than ever, around the quality of our conversations. When we're burnt out or tired, we really feel the impact of words and the quality of a conversation against our tired spirit.

For me, suddenly, every word someone said felt like a slow motion tennis serve, and I could see the spin of the ball coming my way. In the past, conversation just happened, unquestioned and responded to. I would feel uncomfortable or tired but would let the gossip flow on unchallenged or allow trauma dumping. But now, I was catching each word and holding it up to the light, examining its value. I started dropping the words that held gossip, drama, and negativity, and didn't hit them back over the net. I thought, "Don't people think about what they are saying? Don't they consider the constitution of their words?"

I actually stopped a friend mid political tirade and said, "I just can't handle this topic right now, I'm really tired." She just said, "Oh, I get it," and we moved

What If It All Goes Right?

the conversation into something softer and more pleasant.

When we speak with close friends often, there can be a comfortability and informality with topics we launch into, but these days, we have an agreement that drama needs to set an appointment time.

Trauma-dumping without asking permission is like someone stopping by your house, brushing past you standing in the door in your robe, and tossing their trash in the middle of your living room without your permission. They should call first.

When we are with friends going through difficult times, it's nice to carefully curate our words like we are picking flowers, filling the air with something beautiful and worthy and healing.

Boundaries have become one of the most important things in my life. Defining them, setting them, and holding them. It's a practice, and I still struggle. There were a few times that I mysteriously "lost" a cell phone call because I couldn't handle the conversation, and the "End" button was so conveniently located.

Sometimes, the person we need to say "no" to is ourself. I've had to set limits, like avoiding the news when I feel fragile, not dwelling on a fear thought, not gossiping, avoiding sugar, not drinking coffee after a certain time, no electronics two hours before bed, limiting social media, and not overdoing it or getting too busy. I fall short every day, but I am trying.

My dear friend gave me a round red button that says "NO!" in several different ways when you press it. It's one of my favorite things. The word "no" is among the most important and powerful words we use.

> **In Practice**
> - What do you need to say *no* to?
> - What things, situations, invitations, thoughts, or people do you need to put boundaries around?
> - Practice saying no. It's a muscle worth strengthening.
> - What is your time worth and what is worthy of you giving your energy to?

4. Nap Brag: A Call to Inaction

"Doing nothing often leads to the very best of something."

—Winnie the Pooh

A few years ago, I remember heading out to get a massage when one of my relatives was visiting. I felt like I was heading off to a bank heist, slinking out my back door to my appointment off to meet up with a stranger. It feels decadent and like a waste of money, to lie down on a table, close my eyes, and listen to Enya, deep breathing lavender essentials oils when there is a world that needs vacuuming.

When we take care of ourselves, we can better take care of others. When we are rested and restored, we are more calm, less quick to anger, and have more patience for our families.

There is an old Scottish word *hurkle-durkle*, which is a term that means to lounge in bed long after it's time to get up. We need to adopt that term into the English language.

Why is it that if we happen to fall asleep unexpectedly during the day and someone calls, that we jolt up, wipe the drool off the side of our mouth, and answer in a perky voice reserved for game show hosts announcing they've just won something? They

Scarlet Keys

ask, "Were you sleeping?" and we say "Oh no!" or "I was just resting my eyes." How about, "Yes, I was taking a nap!" Normalizing self-care.

Overworking is a value upheld in a capitalist society where the first question people ask you is "What do you do?"

My friend from Nashville is a mom of two and had recently earned her Ph.D. in theology and had surgery during my time of treatment. We have had many conversations about the pressure to be producing something and having something worthy to say when someone asks, "What have you been doing lately?" But I had just bought a hammock, and she was forced on the couch to recover, so we started texting one another things like a picture of my toes peeking out from the soft blanket on my hammock underneath my winterberry tree, and she would text "just took a nap," and then I'd text "doing nothing," and it felt like two Buddhists being competitive to see who could do the most nothing. We would text "Just reading," or "Just watched a bee flit from flower to flower!" or "Just lying here."

We need a self-care revolution where we post on Instagram: "I'm struggling today, so I walked on the beach or met up with a friend and had the best conversation. Sat and read. Slept 'til noon."

Change is difficult and I have to practice staying in the middle lane because my alignment gets off and I veer back into the fast lane. As I have slowed down and focused on healing, I still want to do things that bring meaning, like write, and teach, and visit with

What If It All Goes Right?

friends. When I start to notice the first signs of stress (or veering back into the old fast lane) I have found that I have stress about having stress. I am working on learning how to do nothing, and I feel like people expect to find me wrapped in bubble-wrap, sipping on green juice. They will find me busy but taking time to rest.

I am learning what self-care and healing look like. The middle way is a daily practice.

We need better questions than "What did you do today" or "What do you do?"

How about: "What *didn't* you do today?" Or "did you do anything fun today?" Or "What did you do today to take care of yourself?"

The world won't give us rest, we have to ask for it or take it.

Let's do more of what the world considers to be nothing, and then brag about it. Things like napping, drawing, making art, gardening, baking a lavender cake, writing an old friend a card or letter, watching cat videos, dancing in the kitchen, laughing, sitting quietly, or reading by the ocean. Having nothing to show for our time frivolously spent with beautiful empty hours.

In Practice

- Schedule a little down time each day, even ten minutes.
- Take up a new hobby.
- Do something silly and fun.
- Sleep in late once a week.
- Book an appointment for a massage or something that will relax you.
- Just sit.

5. What Would Henry Do?

"Our life is frittered away by detail. Simplify, simplify, simplify! I say, let your affairs be as two or three, and not a hundred or a thousand; instead of a million count half a dozen, and keep your accounts on your thumb-nail."

—Henry David Thoreau

There is a story about Henry David Thoreau writing Ralph Waldo Emerson a letter that said "Our life is frittered away with detail. Simplify, simplify, simplify." In response, Emerson replied, "One 'simplify' would have sufficed." In his book *Walden*, Thoreau writes, "The cost of a thing, is the amount of what I will call life which is required to be exchanged for it, immediately or in the long run."

I remember walking through the Sleepy Hollow cemetery in Concord Massachusetts where Thoreau is buried, looking for his grave. I passed large and elaborate shrines and monuments and when I finally found where Thoreau was buried, there was only a small headstone set low in the ground with just one word inscribed; it simple said "Henry." I smiled at the integrity of the man who built a small cabin near Walden to be with nature in solitude because he "wished to live deliberately."

Scarlet Keys

Live deliberately. Examining what matters, what matters most, and what doesn't or no longer matters. Some things matter; they hold a memory or sentimentality to them because of what they signify. But so much of what we carry and own is just stuff. Stuff we move around, walk around, feel stressed by, or use our precious hours cleaning or repairing.

I know there is truth in the axiom "Cluttered house, cluttered mind," and that clutter causes anxiety. I wanted to lighten my load and live in a beautiful and clean house where things were easy to find and calming to live with. After Marie Kondo made the whole world self-conscious for owning too many things, I took stock of the things I owned: things in boxes, in the garage, and the basement, in my mind, and I often ask, "What would Henry do?"

I wanted to stop using words like *foraging* and *search party* when looking for my keys or wallet. It was time for a place for everything and everything in its place. I wanted to get rid of things I hadn't used in years, giving up the hope of all jeans size 8 and lower and the army of mismatched coffee cups and Tupperware lids. I gave up my delusion of finding the missing socks, and I renamed my "junk" drawer.

There is also mental clutter. So, I love the idea that an uncluttered room leads to an uncluttered mind, and do find that I think and work better when my environment is clean and organized. Mental clutter can include old resentments, negative thought patterns, or emotional habits that no longer serve us. We can line up the people in our life and note the

What If It All Goes Right?

quality of each relationship. Energy vampires and drama mama's might not make the cut.

Worry, fear, jealousy, negative self-talk, and certain people and activities are as important to stuff in a garbage bag to be donated as the sequined go-go shorts you were never meant to wear.

I am also working on simplifying the plan, the day, and the vacation. If there's an easier way to do things, I'll take the easy way. And I don't feel like I have to go to the party or the book club or fly to Italy to feel like life is fabulous. I no longer have FOMO (fear of missing out) now; I have JOMO (*joy* of missing out) and laugh remembering how many times my dad would say "Do yourself a favor, act like you did, and don't."

We may not be willing to live in a 10 by 15 foot cabin, like Thoreau, but we can simplify. Now, when I have the urge to buy something new that I don't really need, or can't part with an old sweater, or a worn out belief, I stop and ask, "What would Henry do?"

In Practice

- Donate things you have kept out of obligation or that you no longer use.
- Hire a cleaner or ask for help to clean your house. It feels good to live in a simple and clean space.
- Say "no" to things in order to simplify your day or your life. Instead of shopping for a gift, send flowers. Instead of traveling, go someplace local or have a staycation. If you're tired, cancel plans, etc. Easy does it.
- Take a life inventory of things, thoughts, plans, and people in your life. Consider how they affect the quality of your life. Let go of who and what no longer supports your happiness and health.

6. Being Your Own Bodyguard

"The First Wealth is Health."
—Ralph Waldo Emerson

Our body isn't along for the ride. Our body is the vehicle, and we need to take care of it.

I knew I couldn't get well in the same life I got sick in. I knew I had to take a look at how I was living.

There were so many days I just pushed through. If I was tired, I would drink a cup of coffee. I would teach a class and run to the next one without any time in between. I rarely sat down to take a break and put everyone else's needs before my own.

My body had been along for the ride, and it was time to take good care of myself so that I could stick around and be here for the people I loved.

I started to take inventory of my daily activities, breaking down the way I lived and the choices I was making.

I noted that I talk on the phone on my long commute to and from work, and I didn't realize how much I was taxing my mind while navigating traffic, while trying to be a good listener. Then, I would try to find parking in Boston, which should be officially considered for a new Olympic sport, and then I would go straight to teaching all day eating meals on the go.

Working all day wasn't working for me anymore. When I got home, I felt like a rock star coming down from a concert. I was wound up and would want to watch TV and eat a trough of popcorn just to decompress.

It's wonderful to be creative and to have passion projects, but I am now trying to figure out how to be busy and productive without being stressed and having it adversely affect my health.

I ask myself the following questions: How do I wake up? What is the first thought I have in the morning? How could I create a routine that would set me up better than scrolling Instagram and drinking coffee and rushing out the door?

When do I allow myself downtime, and what can I do to restore myself so I can have this productive and rich life I love?

I need to live better and am determined to change the way I live in order to take care of this body so that it will take care of me.

I aim to have a morning routine. to begin each day by saying "I love you" to myself. I say a short list of meditations and a prayer, and I name a few things that I'm grateful for. Sometimes, I play my favorite song to prime myself for the day I want to have. On the days that I start by scrolling social media or am late somewhere, I forgive myself and aim to do things that will steer me towards wellness for the rest of the day and start again tomorrow.

What If It All Goes Right?

I try not to talk on the phone while driving. I try to just drive. That's enough.

Being late is a result of poor time management, and the concept of "transitional stress" is real. I had to notice how I felt as I go from place to place and how I transition from one thing to another.

I try to leave early, so I can arrive early. Just arriving early can change our lives and take a heap of stress off the day.

I take my breaks, and I make it a goal to take short breaks in the day where I can just sit and breathe even for five minutes or do a short, guided meditation to reset.

I used to jump in the car right after work, but now, I try to take a walk, have a conversation with a work colleague, or meditate before jumping into traffic.

I am changing the way I think about a lifetime of eating. We often think of food for how what we eat will make us look or how Ben and Jerry's Chocolate Chip Cookie Dough can make a hard day feel better. Then, as a parent, it might be that we eat so we can have a little more energy to get through the day instead of resting. Now, when I eat or drink something, I think about how it will or won't nourish me, how it will make me feel, and if it is in service of health. I write this while digesting chocolate-chip cookies, but it's progress, not perfection, and there is kale in my near future.

Now, when I feel tired, I rest. When I am around a conversation or person who feels toxic, I try to remove myself from the conversation or situation that is draining my energy. I am my own bodyguard.

When I am presented with a request, a project, or an invitation, and my entire body recoils in horror at the thought of it, I listen to how it makes my body feel. Then, I decline. I have amends to make to my body, and I hope it can start trusting that I will take better care of her.

What If It All Goes Right?

In Practice

Take an inventory of the way you live by breaking down a day in your life. We usually reflect on what we have accomplished, but in this case, look over your day for evidence of self-care.

Daily Inventory:
- How did you take care of yourself today?
- What were your transitions like?
- Were you early to arrive places?
- How did you start the day?
- Did you exercise?
- Did you find time for enjoyment?
- What made you laugh?
- Did you have a quiet moment for yourself to do nothing?
- What are some stressors you can avoid or change?
- Did you take time to meditate, breathe, or pray?
- What is something you can change about your day that would support a healthy life?

7. The Sound of Quiet

"Listen to Silence, it has so much to say."

—Rumi

Silence is the complete absence of sound and is a high reach in this noisy world. It's a rare commodity found in early light after snowfall, swimming underwater, in an anechoic chamber, or beneath a starry desert sky.

I am aiming for quiet. I find quiet to be a crucial part of healing and restoration, and I seek it out as often as possible, minimizing unnecessary sounds in search of rare air.

When we go through something traumatic, we need to be gentle with ourselves and gentle with our recovering nervous system. Quiet and hushed moments are crucial, and we need to make quiet a priority.

We have to make an effort to find quiet and spend time in it. I am a bit claustrophobic, so I haven't quite found the bravery to book a salt-water float tank, bathing with my own thoughts. Short of renting a submarine or mortgaging my house to fly to space, I am left with settling for less noise.

When I am alone at home, I turn off my phone and my computer and enjoy as much quiet as I can find.

What If It All Goes Right?

Even the sounds of nature count as quiet to me: brushing past lady slipper orchids in the forest, and the chatter of birds. The whisper of wind, and the sound of my breath against my heartbeat. These are sounds that make sense to my soul.

I consider the sounds of the beach to be my kind of quiet. The crackle of the bubbled breath of small waves collapsing on wet sand and seagulls. Or in the Midwest in a vast open field where I can see nothing for miles and miles, and the sound of stillness.

Quiet allows us to tune into our intuition, and is crucial for times when we need to make big decisions or figure out our next right step. Your higher power may be nature, or you might not have a spiritual belief, but to me, God speaks in whispers, and I like to turn down the noise so I can hear.

Quiet is restorative, and for the creative, blank space and boredom allow space for ideas to be born.

In Practice

- Take a ten minute sound break every day where you can spend time in the most quiet space you can find.
- Take time to go outside and listen to only the sounds of nature.

8. The "S" Word

"For a day, just for one day, talk about that which disturbs no one, and bring some peace into your beautiful eyes."

—Hafiz

I used to think the "F" word was the worst word, but have come to find out, it's actually "Stress" that wins the prize.

It is true that stress isn't the problem. It's our reaction to stress that is the problem.

The "S" word creates a bodily stress response by just hearing the word. Oftentimes, what we automatically label "stress" is actually emotional overload or dread or some granular form of the word stress. Maybe it's a scheduling problem, or we need help getting organized and prioritizing our time. Maybe it's a boundary problem, or a lack of taking and protecting down time. Maybe we should prioritize fun.

There is something called the Life Change Index Scale that rates major life events in order of the most stress provoking to the least. Things that rank high are: the death of a spouse, divorce, jail term, the death of a close family member, illness, being fired, and mortgage foreclosure. The list continues.

What If It All Goes Right?

Little things can add up, and life gets messy. There will always be difficult visiting relatives, difficult coworkers, taxes, bills, traffic, and the undercurrent of a global angst we all feel about the state of the world.

Stress can feel like something we own, as in "I have a lot of stress." Or we can embody it, as in "I am so stressed." It can feel like a hard rain coming on out of nowhere. Clothes drenched, day ruined. But stress is not a state; stress is a response.

I am learning to choose my response to people places and things, especially the unwelcome and challenging things.

We can't stop the rain, but we can open our umbrella, run for cover, or marvel at the storm. Or as Eckhart Tolle says, "If you find your here and now intolerable and it makes you unhappy, you have three options: remove yourself from the situation, change it, or accept it totally."

In Practice

- Notice the things that are causing you stress that you have control over.
- Notice self-inflicted stress that is avoidable, such as inviting guests to stay for too long, over-volunteering, listening to too many people unload their problems, or saying yes to doing things that you really don't want to do.

9. Antidotes to Stress

"Guard well your spare moments. They are like uncut diamonds. Discard them and their value will never be known. Improve them and they will become the brightest gems in a useful life."

—Ralph Waldo Emerson

Here are some tools that I have found really useful as antidotes to stress.

Humor

Humor is magical at changing a moment. Laughter is medicine, and if you've ever been on the tipping point of a fight and then all of a sudden ended up folded over in incurable laughter at your absurdity, you know the life-changing effects of laughter. Humor is becoming my moment-to-moment goal, and it has diffused countless stress-provoking moments in my day-to-day.

I recently went shopping with my daughter and asked her to carry in the trash from the car. She asked me to do it. I said my hands were full and that she should carry it in. And then our tone of voices got tighter and more irritated as she pushed for me to take it. I felt my irritation beginning to flare, so I said in a squeaky Kim Kardashian voice, "You're making this so hard," and we both laughed, and dissolved some of the tension.

Instead of anger at a car cutting us off in traffic, we make up funny stories about why that driver is in such a hurry. Maybe he has debilitating diarrhea, or he peaked in high school, or there's a bee in his car.

Listening to stand-up comedy in traffic is a good one too.

Scheduling

So much overwhelm can be avoided by the choices we make and how we plan our day, our week, and our month. It's important not to over schedule our time. I am becoming very mindful of how much I plan during a day and throughout the week and make sure I take breaks and create margins in the day to just sit, meditate, breathe, or take a walk.

Breath Work

Breath work isn't new but is now widely practiced for its health benefits and for stress reduction. There are many forms of breath work to choose from and I encourage you to explore a practice that works for you. Breath work is a portable tool we can use anytime or place to calm our nervous system. Here are two techniques you can try:

- 4-7-8: Breathe in for four counts, hold your breath for seven counts, and then exhale for eight counts.
- Deep abdominal breathing: Take a long deep breath. As you breathe in, imagine the

air is filling your body. Your chest and belly expand with each inhale. Exhale until you can feel your navel move towards and almost touch your spine. When we breathe like this, we tell our body to relax.

Focusing on our breathing gives our bodies time to recover from the effects of stress and time to reset.

Get Moving

Once the body feels anxious and the amygdala is ringing its bell, we can't think our way out of it. We need to metabolize the stress. The problem now belongs to the body with its fear or dread. There is accumulated stress that we hold at the end of each day. We can metabolize the adrenaline and cortisol by walking, constricting and releasing our muscles, and if possible, doing planks, or shaking to release negative feelings in the body. You might like dancing, running, or gardening. Anything that moves us moves our emotions.

Mindfulness and Meditation

I've been trying to make meditation a daily habit. My meditation teacher has helped me stay on track living a healthier life.

When we had a session about stress, he worked with me on changing ownership of stress from "I am stressed out" to "I am feeling stress."

"A part of me is experiencing stress right now but part of me isn't."

This idea is so helpful in shrinking difficult

emotions down to their proper size. I can then expand the part of me that isn't feeling stressed.

Mindfulness, for me, requires that I do one thing at a time. It turns out that our brains weren't meant for multitasking. It's a myth, it's stressful, and we don't get the best results from anything we are doing.

I practice mindfulness and being in the moment. This moment is all we really have and are guaranteed. *This* moment, not the next. Eckhart Tolle says, "Unease, anxiety, tension, stress—all forms of fear are caused by too much future and not enough presence." He says, "Wherever you are, be there totally."

Since I have opened up to being willing to try new things in honor of living a healthier life, I made an appointment to learn transcendental meditation at a center in Boston. I received my mantra and have been practicing TM along with guided meditations. At times, it's hard to commit to, but I am trying, and when I do it, I feel so much more resilient, calm, and better able to handle life's challenges.

I try to make meditation a priority for even five minutes a day, if nothing else.

Animals

Animals are such a huge source of love, healing, and calm, to me. When I first got diagnosed, I said to my husband, "I'm going to need a chemo kitten." He said, "No, we don't need another cat," so I said, "or a chemo Mercedes," and he said, "What kind of kitten?"

We adopted our little lanky, squinty-eyed rescue with his broken tail. He was orange and awkward and nervous, so we named him Conan after Conan O'Brien. He would snuggle my left side and stretch his little arms across my chest and purr. It was like he knew which side of me needed healing.

Touch from humans and from pets allows us to co-regulate and borrow their peace. When we experience kind touch, the body releases the bonding hormone oxytocin. This hormone creates feelings of well-being and trust and can be released with exercise, touch, hugs, massage, and singing with others.

At one point, on a very stressful day, I was upstairs in my bedroom. I was leaning against the wall, holding our other cat Pam, and desperately breathing deeply into her fur. My husband walked in, and said "Stop inhaling the cat." I burst into laughter, because I realized that she was my oxytocin hostage.

Self-Talk

The things we think and say affect our bodies. I try to be careful of what I think and say because I know that our bodies respond to the quality of our words and thoughts. When I'm having a hard day, I try telling myself things like, "I can do this," or "All is well," or "This too shall pass," or "I've got this." Just saying something comforting to myself helps to calm the moment.

Mindset

How we look at things is so important. Glass half

What If It All Goes Right?

empty or full is a cliché for a reason, and I try to look for the good in every situation.

I have found it very de-stressing to change the statement "I have to" to "I choose to" or "I get to."

Even saying "I get to go to the dentist" is empowering and infused with gratitude at the opportunity to have such a miraculous option.

I would go to chemotherapy, and when the nurse would leave the room after hanging my IV bag up on the hook of the pole, I would stand up and draw a heart on the bag of taxol and send a little thank you to the yew tree where they discovered the medicine that was healing me.

In Practice

- Seek out laughter. Listen to stand-up comedy or watch funny videos. Make an effort to lighten up and look for the humor in things. Spend time with people who make you laugh.
- Protect your time and energy by taking the time to schedule your day and week or month.
- Practice some form of breath work each day.
- Practice mindfulness and being in the moment.
- Limit watching the news and social media.
- Exercise at least 30 minutes a day.
- Meditate at least 10 minutes a day.
- Watch the quality of your thoughts and conversations.
- Practice optimism.

10. Joy

"Find ecstasy in life; the mere sense of living is joy enough."

—Emily Dickinson

Happiness is fickle and transient. Happiness can be an impossible ask in the darkest times. But if happiness and savoring had a child, they would name her Joy.

Joy is reliable and can be found on our darkest day. Joy holds meaning and is wider and deeper than happiness. Joy is an inner feeling that can appear while enduring hardships and is imbued with meaning and purpose. Joy is one of the highest vibrational emotions we can experience. It's a wonderful state to be in for healing and recovery and can be found through the cracks in the darkest day.

Joy is often associated with roller-coasters and Disneyland. But as an adult, it doesn't have to be *Joy* with a capital J. It can be softer and subtler, with a lowercase j contained in words like *joyful* or *enjoyment*.

Joy is a spectrum emotion from fireflies to fireworks, and on hard days, I aim for fireflies. Emotions like bliss, glee, and elation feel impossible, so I settle into delight, gladness, and comfort. On some days, I revel in the simple joy of being wrapped in a favorite blanket and listening to a song.

What If It All Goes Right?

I have found that I don't have to do the big things, I can find enjoyment in reading a good book, learning something new, sitting by the ocean, working in my garden, writing a song, or just organizing my house and making it more beautiful. I am aiming for joyful.

My father had been in the ICU for thirty days. He was eighty years old, and his life was touch and go. His skin was so thin and fragile that the nurses had taped his arms, and he was bruised and tired. I remember, one day his bed was facing the window, and he looked at me and said "This was the most wonderful day." And I said, "Dad, you're in ICU, and I just suctioned your spit," and he said "I'm here with you, we can see the beautiful sunset out the window, and I've got all these crazy broads running around bringing me things." It made me laugh in wonderment, how this man was finding something beautiful in that beige room in such uncertain times.

When we look around us during our most challenging times, finding joy reminds us there is magic in the world. Finding joy is an actionable and worthy endeavor and can be found even in a hospital room.

There are times when going out joy hunting isn't practical or possible, but we can borrow it from a memory. Closing our eyes, placing our hands on our heart, and casting our memory back to a joyful time or a moment that filled us with joy. Memories hold joy for us ready to be retrieved and felt again when it's hard to find in the moment we are in.

Scarlet Keys

We can look for tiny beautiful things, comforting things, a flower, kindness from a stranger or a friend, our cat purring on our chest, a soft blanket, an unexpected laugh, the touch of a loved one, or listening to a favorite piece of music or a song. Just one small beautiful thing savored can activate joy, and we can reach for them when things are hard.

Some of my big "J" joys have included walking into the Dominican convent of Santa Maria delle Grazie one day in Milan, with my best friend, when no one else was there, and staring up at da Vinci's painting of the last supper. Swimming with a dolphin, seeing Barbra Streisand in concert. Then there is a higher form of joy, elation, such as the birth of my daughter or falling in love with my husband.

As a practice, it's good for our health to aim for the highest form of joy. It's good for our mood and our immune system. So go for a joyride with a blaze in your heart.

What brings you joy? Maybe right now it's joy with a lower case "j": a cup of tea and the feel of your favorite mug in your hands, or playing or learning an instrument, making art, helping others, praying, or recalling sweet memories.

When we have the energy, we can reach a little higher on the spectrum, like riding a horse, or going to an arcade, or drinking coffee on a swing, or skipping down the street. Or we might go to a concert, fly to a new destination, take a salsa lesson, or dive into a summer wave.

In Practice

- What brings you joy?
- Each day, try to find something that brings you joy, not matter how small or simple.
- End your day recounting the things that brought you joy that day. It's a wonderful feeling to take into your sleep with you.

11. The Self-Love Club

"You can search throughout the entire universe for someone who is more deserving of your love and affection than you are yourself, and that person is not to be found anywhere. You yourself, as much as anybody in the entire universe deserve your love and affection."

—Buddha

I have had an on-again/off-again relationship with myself most of my life and often let fluctuating numbers affect how I feel about myself. The number on the scale, the balance of my bank account, the number of wrinkles, and my age.

But with age and experience, I have turned towards the numbers that really count, like how many true friends I have, how many moments that take my breath away, how many times I've laughed folded over and breathless, the countries I've visited, the good things I've done, and sometimes, my blood count.

Life is short, and we don't have the luxury of spending one more minute trying to win ourselves over. Not one more minute trying to convince ourselves that we are worthy of our own love or that we are good enough. What does good enough even mean?

What If It All Goes Right?

So much of how we feel about ourselves is based on comparing our lives with someone else's, and I love the Teddy Roosevelt quote, "Comparison is the thief of joy."

I make my husband laugh when I call another driver an ass hat in traffic and then I feel bad and say, "Mother Theresa would never have said that." He will then say, "So that's your gauge? A saint?"

I'm either feeling that I've done nothing in a day because Oprah has a magazine, an Oscar, and a school for girls in Africa, or like a glutton because Gandhi would have never eaten that whole thing."

If we are going to compare ourselves, why don't we do ourselves a favor and aim lower, because compared to Attila the Hun and jay walkers, I'm actually not that bad.

We all fall on the spectrum of good and bad. We are just weird humans made of stardust and insecurity, spinning through space on a random planet, doing our best even when our best is our worst and we need grace and forgiveness over and over again.

Perfection is a ridiculous ideal and can't be measured. All I know is that no one wants to be around anyone who is perfect, and as far as I'm concerned, my friends are all a little relieved when we have a reunion, and we are all just a little bit pudgier with a few more grey hairs.

People only post their filtered highlights on social media, not their lowlights. We are all we've got, and we need be our own cheerleader and our own best friend.

Scarlet Keys

When we've gone through a health crisis, we abandon the ridiculous dream of thigh gap and adopt an appreciation not for what our body looks like but for what it does for us. It can all come down to being grateful to be able to walk and thanking our strong hearts for continuing to beat.

What a shame, to take our one and only one-of-a-kind self and grimace in the mirror, scanning for imperfections, and handing the mean critic the mic.

Self-love is a practice. It works better as an action than a concept, and it's a daily habit built from doing estimable acts, and practicing self-compassion. Being gentle with our humanness. It's built of taking care of ourselves the way we would take care of someone we love.

Eating well, exercising, making the bed, planning ahead, not torturing ourselves with reading mean comments or beating ourselves up for blunders. Being honest, nurturing the things that make us happy, and forgiving the younger version of ourselves who got us here—however flawed they were.

Sometimes, self-love can be as simple as making the decision to love yourself. One day, I just decided to stand up tall, shoulders back, head held high, shaking off the past like snow on a coat, and said, "Hey you flawed but wonderful woman, you with the jowls and the crepe skin, yes you. You with your nice legs and good hair, you who are doing your best, yes, you: I love you."

Then I said "I am so sorry I made you wait so long and work so hard to win the love of the only person worthy and qualified to love you." And I said it not in the voice of Regina George but in the voice of the fairy Godmother.

What If It All Goes Right?

In Practice

Self-love in action:

1. Find a picture of yourself before the age of ten, and take a photo of it to keep on your phone or print it out, and have it next to your bed or bathroom mirror.
2. Every morning look at that little version of you, and send them love.
3. Look in the mirror for even thirty seconds a day and say, "I love you."
4. Make a list of ways you could treat yourself like someone who is deserving of love.

Some things to consider:

- Eat veggies.
- Say no.
- Say yes.
- Be honest.
- Dress your best.
- Be organized.
- Exercise.
- Talk to yourself in a kind voice.
- Forgive yourself.
- Make your bed.
- Arrive everywhere early.
- Don't procrastinate. (It's mean to give your future self an entire sink of dishes or pile of bills.)
- Think well of yourself.
- Wear a tiara while you vacuum (you'd be surprised).
- Forgive yourself when you fall short of all of these suggestions.

12. Nature

"Live in the Sunshine, Swim the Sea, Drink the wild air."

—Ralph Waldo Emerson

It turns out the "tree huggers" were on to something.

We have gotten so far away from nature as a society that we often go weeks without touching the ground with our bare feet.

So many of us live in cities or work at companies where we are inside most of the day. We sit in front of computers beneath florescent lights and then walk down concrete streets to our cars or subways and then back home to our TVs and Wi-Fi.

I started meeting with a woman on Zoom once a week who I called my vibe coach. One of the things she encouraged me to do was to take my shoes off and put my bare feet on the ground for thirty minutes a day to boost my immune system.

In honor of practicing hope, I was staying open to trying anything that would be helpful and healing, including starting with a daily habit of sitting in my garden to work outside with my shoes off and feel the soft grass beneath my feet.

What If It All Goes Right?

I felt calmer and more peaceful, barefoot among the flowers and trees. I also made time for more barefoot beach walks, and started to crave nature.

"Grounding" or "Earthing" has been practiced for centuries. The concept of connecting to the earth's natural electrical charge has been used by ancient cultures for both healing and spiritual purposes for thousands of years.

Oncologist Leigh Erin Connealy talks about the potential health benefits of grounding, saying it causes a reduction in inflammation, helps with sleep and stress, boosts our immune system, and can help accelerate wound healing.

Soil microbes have been found to have similar effects on the brain as antidepressants. The bacterium may stimulate serotonin production, which makes us relaxed and happier.

In Japan, the practice of forest bathing or forest therapy (or shinrin-yoku) is not just walking in the woods, but being mindful. Luxuriating in and engaging our senses. There is a chemical that trees and plants emit called *phytoncides*, which are considered to be the medicine of the forest.

Phytoncides are tree essential oils that have many medicinal purposes. The chemicals given off by trees contain antimicrobial and insecticidal qualities that protect the trees from parasites and germs. When we breathe in these chemicals, our bodies respond by increasing the number of and activity of white blood cells, called natural killer cells.

Scarlet Keys

Trees emit active substances and create a field of protection around them against harmful bugs, bacteria, and disease. By just walking near them, we can reap the benefit of much more than just their oxygen. Scientists say that just looking at the color green increases feelings of well-being, and that walking in a forest for two hours can boost natural killer cells for two weeks after time spent in the forest.

Emerson said, "When I go into my garden with a spade, and dig a bed, I feel such an exhilaration and health that I discover that I have been defrauding myself all this time in letting others do for me what I should have done with my own hands."

I always feel more relaxed when I have spent time in nature, and especially in my own garden, digging in the soil.

In Practice

- How can you spend more time in nature?
- Can you work outside?
- Take your shoes off and touch the ground during your lunch hour or break? Work in the garden without gloves on, or sit in a garden and work or read?
- Take a forest walk or find a tree lined street in your neighborhood. Spend a little time in nature every day.
- Take a few minutes every day to go outside and look up. Take a few deep breaths.

13. Hard Gifts

"Barn's burnt down—now I can see the moon."
—Mizuta Masahide

When we face the hardest things, we shed the superficial and the material, and life is stripped down to the essentials and what matters most.

When I first told my brother about the treatment I was about to face, he said, "This will make you stronger." My reaction was, "Who cares about being stronger!" I am strong enough. I know he meant well, but yuck, what a prize to endure. I get to be stronger?

There are things that only come from the hardest things. Not everything we gain feels like a blessing or a gift. Some things are bittersweet and hard-earned, like medals from war. Some sort of broken beauty that comes from adversity.

There are amazing things that come from hard things, like valleys carved from rivers, or desert dunes from winds that have blown for hundreds of years. Great trees from acorns, the pyramids, the six hundred years it took to build the Gothic Cologne Cathedral, 1 to 3.3 billion years to form a diamond, or six months for an oyster to make a pearl. The nine months of pregnancy, then the hard labor, and then your child in your arms. The hardest break of the bad goodbye and then a new love, the diploma in hand and the pride in the graduate's smile, the high after the marathon, or the relief of surviving the dive from the airplane. Malcolm Gladwell's ten thousand hours of practice to become an expert or months to years in becoming a warrior after enduring a long divorce, recovery, or health challenge.

Some gifts are harder won than others, and some feel unwelcome or not worth the cost. Even within the worst things we face and overcome, we can always find meaning. And we earn the unseen prizes of strength: knowing how brave we can be, a feeling of pride, and amazement to know what we are really made of.

One of the hardest things for me was holding my grandmother's hand in the hospital as she slipped from this world. It was hard for me, but it was meaningful to be there with her in that moment. Years later, my brother and I stood on either side of my father's hospital bed saying "I love you" over and over again as our favorite person took his last breath. These hard things give us the strength to serve others.

A dear friend of ours recently passed away, and my husband and I dove head-first into the last months of his life with him because we had a strength that was hard-won and was now in service of someone needing his friends to come in closer than ever, as he was living his last days. That was hard, because we got so close to him and then had to say goodbye.

What If It All Goes Right?

We always keep the love we give and in the hardest moments of our lives, we are never left empty-handed. There is always a parting gift.

I haven't searched for gifts from my rubble as much as I have found them. I didn't know I could live deeper and wider, and more fearlessly. I love better and more fully, I'm kinder, and I'm more honest. I am bitchier when needed, I'm less of a people-pleaser, and I swear more. I am trying to only do the things I really want to do or spend time with people I cherish. I have reconnected with distant family members and scattered friends. The past few years are still teaching me, and it has all led to my writing this book.

As it turns out, I am stronger, and although I didn't want to be, I bring that strength with me to the side of other people facing hard things, saying, "You've got this, we've got this!"

In Practice

- What are some of your hard gifts?
- What have you learned from the most challenging things about yourself?
- Close your eyes, and imagine the best possible outcome for any current challenge you are facing. Notice how that feels, and now practice staying in that feeling state.

14. Good Vibes Only

"Hurt feelings don't vanish on their own. They don't heal themselves. If we don't express our emotions, they pile up like a debt that will eventually come due."

—Marc Bracket, Ph.D.

I grew up in southern California where sunny days come with sunny expectations and dispositions and the constant pressure to "Have a great day." I think California must have invented the smiley face. The word *awesome*, which should be reserved for things like the birth of a child or the second coming, is thrown around on everything from your frozen yogurt to the cheese on your nachos—all equally totally awesome! The ideology of "good vibes only" can translate into toxic positivity.

I advocate facing and feeling our emotions but optimism becomes my North Star of emotion to aim towards when negativity becomes my default.

We humans don't come with a feelings manual, and many of us grow up emotionally illiterate, suppressed, or limited. We may have grown up around well-meaning people who don't want us hurting, so they try to make us feel better with a joke or distraction. But their well-meaning attempt to save

What If It All Goes Right?

us from a difficult emotion is oftentimes stealing a vital experience from us or stopping tears that need to be shed.

There's a difference between drying someone's tears and stopping someone's tears.

Maybe, as children, our parents didn't want us to be feeling anything bad or hard or weird, so they interrupted the first sign of upset like they were pulling us away from a hot stove. It could have also been because it's a reflection on their parenting, and what they might be doing to cause an anxious or depressed kid so they brush it off by saying things like, "Oh, don't be scared," or "That's silly/ridiculous," or "What do you have to be anxious about?"—or worse, "Don't be so dramatic," or "Lighten up."

Oftentimes, when we are drenched in hard feelings, people try to change the channel, because if they let *us* have this feeling, they might have to feel *their* feelings. This could trigger their sadness or grief or fear, so they shut it down.

Feelings are here for a reason, and our emotions are a huge part of being human. It's vital that we feel our feelings whatever they are, and that we find healthy ways to process them, regulate them, and learn what they are here to teach us.

I've learned that it's important to express my hard emotions with people who can sit with me—who don't try to change the weather in the room, and can be with whatever is. We need to name it to tame it, as Dr. Daniel Siegel talks about in his book *The Whole-Brain Child*. The irrational part of our brain might be in fear. But if our two brain hemispheres can make meaning out of a feeling, we are better able to calm down.

When my daughter was little, she was scared of monsters under her bed. Instead of instinctively trying to save her from her feelings with, "Oh honey, there is no such thing as monsters," or "Don't be scared, there's nothing to be afraid of," I took a moment to acknowledge her reality starting with, "That must feel really scary, I used to be afraid of monsters under my bed too. That must feel really hard and you're all alone in your room." Then, I'd look under the bed with her and shine a light." Her little self would then feel seen and heard, and she would relax and be able to move forward. Sometimes, we'd find a new way to look at it too by talking about the cute monsters and what if *we* scare *them*, and what if they are really, really cute? And we would usually end up laughing, but first, we gave name to the feelings. When parents say things like, "You shouldn't feel that way" or "There's nothing to be scared of," it gaslights a child's reality, and they may start to feel like their feelings are wrong or bad.

In early childhood education, I remember being given four choices to identify our feelings:

Mad, Glad, Scared, Sad

I'm happy to see that we've added a bit more nuance with: Tired, Calm, Worried, Confused, Silly, Loved, Embarrassed....

In sociology professor Brené Brown's work, she and her team found that on average, people can identify only three emotions as they are actually

What If It All Goes Right?

feeling them: Happiness, Sadness, and Anger. And being able to precisely name our feelings is a crucial skill for knowing ourselves and for connecting with others. According to her work, we have eighty-seven different emotions.

In Dr. Marc Brackett's book *Permission to Feel*, he distinguishes between emotions, feelings, and moods:

Emotions: Automatic, short-lived, response, constructed from previous experiences

Feelings: Internal response to emotion

Moods: Prolonged, where you spend the majority of the time

There's a difference between a feeling and a mood. We need to honor and name our feelings, and decide which ones to name, feel, and express and which ones we don't need to marinate in.

It's vital that we honor whatever feeling we are having, because our feelings are helpful for us to understand our lives. All a feeling wants is to be felt.

It's important to differentiate between the emotions we *need* to experience and the emotions that we *choose* to experience. Pain is part of life, but suffering is a plan. Emotions are important and have something to teach us, so learning to feel them for the appropriate amount of time—as opposed to wallowing or steeping in them—is the challenge.

No matter what the moment holds for us—no matter how scary or hard or even boring—we can choose our response.

Scarlet Keys

As a songwriter and a songwriting professor, I spend a lot of my time with emotions. Expressing them, feeling them, and using music to support them.

For example, we songwriters can compare our own emotional language of Happy, Sad, Mad, Scared to the basic chords in a major key: the three major chords could be considered "happy" sounding, and the three minor chords could be considered "sad."

But when we think of more granular emotions, like lonely or hopeless or nervous or inspired, we think of granular harmony and chords outside of the key we are in, to better support these more nuanced emotions. So now, we have chords that offer more nuanced feelings that can support more nuanced emotion.

For any musicians reading this, we can use the expected chords in a key or borrowed chords. For example, in the key of C major, the chords that support sadness would usually be A minor, D minor and E minor. But when we need to express more nuanced emotions in the category of sadness, we might play an Fmin6 chord or even F#dim to support a more clearly defined emotion of loneliness or the devastation of unrequited love. We could move in the direction of positive chords that support happiness such as F major or G major and then reach for a brighter chord from another key to turn up the volume by using a chord such as D major or E major to express the granular positive emotions that chords provide going from happy to ecstatic or blissful.

What If It All Goes Right?

> **In Practice**
>
> Some ways to increase our emotional awareness:
> - Expand your emotional vocabulary, and become more granular with how you feel.
> - Feel what you are feeling.
> - Cry, if you need to.
> - Write a letter or email you'll never send.
> - Write a song.
> - Journal.
> - Meditate.
> - Talk to a good friend.

15. Words Matter

"The happiness of your life depends on the quality of your thoughts."

—Marcus Aurelius

You can learn a lot about your life by noting your vocabulary. I have taken up swearing like a sixth grader who just learned how. It feels honest, and it feels like I release stress with each expletive, so I think it might be here to freakin' stay.

One of the things I have been doing in my life overhaul is taking an inventory of the words I use consistently. Our lexicon can tell us so much about our emotional life.

What do we say when we talk to ourselves? When we look in the mirror? When we step on the scale or check social media comments?

Words matter.

We think about 70,000 thoughts per day, and 90 percent of the thoughts we think today are the same thoughts we thought yesterday. They go on unquestioned, and we go along with them and believe them. Thoughts that scare us, anger us, cast doubt. Thoughts we chew on, marinate in, and choose again and again.

What If It All Goes Right?

We all have automatic negative thoughts. But more than ever, I have been learning to separate myself from my thoughts a bit more, and to catch any mean or fearful thought and consciously turn it toward something productive, hopeful, funny, or even beautiful.

It's important to consider our thought life, watching and curating the quality of the thoughts we think. One of the most valuable things I've come to know is that thoughts are just thoughts, and just because we *think* something doesn't mean it's true. I've learned to question my thoughts, and I often refer to the work of author Byron Katie, asking myself "Is this thought true?" "Is it helpful?" and "How would I act and feel without this thought?" I also make fun of the crazy or fearful ones.

So many thoughts are useless and sabotaging, especially the things that follow the statement "I am...." I try to be careful how I finish that sentence and catch a thought that no longer serves me.

I remember one day in treatment, one of the nurses came in to check to see if my infusion was complete, and there was a little bit of Taxol left in the bag. She squeezed the bag and said, "Let's see if we can get the last drops of poison in you."

I was horrified. I was in a suggestive and vulnerable state, and quickly said, "I don't call it that, it's my medicine, and I'm grateful for it." I later called the clinic, told them what she said and told them I never wanted her to be my nurse again.

Scarlet Keys

I was so conscious of other people's words and took a long look at my frequented words.

Before my health diagnosis, I commonly used words like:

overwhelmed	*exhausted*	*stressed*	*powering out*
pushing	*hurrying*	*rushed*	*deadline*
pressure	*anxious*	*tired*	*tense*
late			

How did you feel reading that list?
Then we have internal critique words like:

fat	*stupid*	*untalented*	*imposter*
incapable	*lazy*	*messy*	*etc.*

How do you feel when you read that list?

I knew I had to create a life where the byproduct of my daily thoughts and actions created a different list of words. such as:

early	*on time*	*rested*	*relaxed*
present	*easy*	*prepared*	

And then another internal list:

worthy	*loved*	*enough*	*trying*
capable	*deserving*	*doing my best*	

How different did you feel reading this list?

What If It All Goes Right?

I have had to admit that although I grew up with wonderful parents, I also grew up around chaos, and I am working on changing how comfortable I am with chaos.

I have an affirmation I use:
Ease and flow feel like home.

It's my emotional mission statement, and everything I do and think aim to support that self concept.

I have to get comfortable with less cortisol and adrenaline. I practice arriving early and being calm. It is all new neural pathways I am creating in my brain, and retraining my nervous system is a daily and sometimes moment-to-moment process.

I am also very, very careful of what I say after I say "I am." I no longer allow the mean voice to have its say. I stop it mid insult or criticism, and I substitute something healing, supportive, and loving in its place. From "I am so disorganized" to "I am doing my best and will tackle this pile for five minutes." Or "I am ____ [anything negative]" to something that is kind to myself.

I love this bible passage:

> *"Finally, brothers and sisters, whatever is true, whatever is noble, whatever is right, whatever is pure, whatever is lovely, whatever is admirable, if anything is excellent or praise worthy, think about such things."*
>
> —Philippians 4:8

In Practice

- What new mantra could you write for your life?
- Notice what words you most commonly use.
- Notice the quality of your thoughts and words.
- Notice the quality of the conversations you have with others.
- Make a list of words that inspire you or make you feel stronger, and start using more of them.

16. The "F" Word

"When you look fear in the face, you are able to say to yourself, 'I lived through this horror, I can take the next thing that comes along.'"

—Eleanor Roosevelt

"F-E-A-R" has two meanings: *Forget Everything and Run* or *Face Everything and Rise*, according to author/motivational speaker Zig Ziglar, or in my case, *Face Everything Scared and Collect All the Things*, like Steve Martin at the end of the movie *The Jerk*, where I walk into the hard things saying, "All I need is this soft blanket, and this rose quartz, and this lavender spritzer, and that's all… well, and maybe this cozy blanket, and that's all, except for my Wonder Woman key chain and my list of funny cat videos, that's all I need…."

My father grew up during the Great Depression and was in the United States Army in WWII under General George Patton. So, fear and worry weren't anything he showed signs of while I was growing up, because he had faced such hard things.

I grew up in southern California with the threat that we could have the big earthquake and plunge into the ocean any minute. One day, I asked my dad if he ever worries about the big quake and he said,

"Sure, but, I'm not going to start shaking now." I burst out laughing but I never forgot that.

We all wrestle with worry because it's our nature, and we all have fear—whether it's big F Fear or little f fear. From the fear of public speaking to having to confront a hard conversation to leaving a marriage to facing open heart surgery, fear is a part of life. This all takes strength: but we have an inherent strength of spirit and a will to fight and face challenges.

Mark Twain said, "I am an old man and have known a great many troubles, but most of them never happened. Worrying is like paying a debt you don't owe. I have spent most of my life worrying about things that have never happened." I love that, because how much of the worst is just dark imagination before it even happens? I try to be afraid at the moment the scary thing shows up and not waste the three weeks leading up to it. Or as Shakespeare put it, "A coward dies a thousand times before his death, but the valiant taste of death but once." Or as Charlie Keys said, "Don't start shaking now."

There is a relief that comes from avoidance, but there is a strength that comes from facing hard things. I would say that most hard things involve fear and worry, but we can be mindful of it and catch it before we are steeped in dread and turn our thoughts to something higher like prayer, positive imagery, or gratitude. I am still afraid, but at least now, I don't pour my gasoline thoughts on my fear, making it bigger and out of control. I control my part of fear, and I accept that it's going to be part of a big brave

What If It All Goes Right?

life of trying things that make me feel vulnerable (like writing this book).

I want the feeling of bravery over the momentary relief of putting something off or avoiding it. But there are days when we just can't, and I do have those days and that's okay.

One of the things I've heard people say most often to me over the past couple of years is "You're so brave." I didn't see it that way. I felt like I was just doing what needed to be done, like running through fire to get out of the burning house that was falling down around me.

There is a feeling you get after you face something hard that is much higher than the feeling of relief you get from avoiding something. There is a relief to canceling a dental appointment, but there is a strength and pride you get after going in and facing what needs to be done. A feeling that only the brave get to revel in.

Brave is the action we take step by step onto the battlefield or under the wedding canopy, out of the airplane or into the chemo chair.

In Practice

- What is something you've been avoiding due to fear?

- Is there something small you can practice today, like making the appointment? or Sending an email? Or one step towards your dream?

- Think of things you've worried about in the past. How much of what you imagined actually happened? What can you learn from that?

- How can you practice being brave and facing hard things?

17. Altars in the Day

"My altars are the mountains and the ocean."
—Lord Byron

Altars are sacred spiritual spaces—places to reflect and often to present an offering. Usually, we think of the objects placed on altars: incense, candles, wine, etc. But in the altar of our heart, we can place mental objects, such as the faces of people we love, things we are grateful for, memories that make us smile, or a chance to meditate on what we want to see expanded in our day or within ourselves, such as kindness, faith, sobriety, hope, or joy.

In a bookstore, I recently witnessed a stranger unfurl their prayer mat and kneel in the middle of the aisle to pray. She was in the writing section of the store where I needed to search for a book. Another girl was sort of standing guard as she claimed a space in the middle of a crowded bookstore for a sacred moment, forehead to floor, in prayer. Her friend respectfully stopped me and said, "She's almost done praying."

So, I waited.

She stood and rolled up her prayer mat. I asked, "Did you have enough time?" and she said, "Yes," and they were on their way.

Scarlet Keys

I was struck by her commitment to her faith and that she had made time and space to create a sacred moment in her day.

I watched a Chinese woman in the Boston Commons practicing her Tai Chi, Christians bowing their heads to say grace at a restaurant, and more and more of my friends and people I know taking time in their day to meditate or spend a little time in prayer.

I search for cracks in the day, on busy days, where I can take time to close my eyes, meditate, or pray. Even if I only have five minutes, I try to close my eyes and breathe, or I will listen to a short guided meditation.

Always at hand is our breath. It is always available to us as a way to find calm and connect to ourselves.

Altars aren't found only in shrines, temples, churches, or other places of worship. We can create an altar wherever we are. More than once, the seat of my car has been a sacred space. A place to practice patience and acceptance on a long commute. It's also become a place to meditate when I'm parked, or to pray, or to take a quick, restorative nap.

We can all find a quiet space during the day—even if it's the bathroom (since that's the only room we can go into alone for an unlimited amount of time with no questions asked), or in our car, or an empty room where we can take a break.

There is an altar in your heart—a traveling resting place that is always available, where you can stop and close your eyes and breathe. A respite from

What If It All Goes Right?

the world or traffic or work, where we take a break from the noise and go within.

In the Robin Williams documentary *Come Inside My Mind*, there was a scene where he was overseas in Iraq and Afghanistan on a U.S.O. tour with comedian Lewis Black, giving every ounce of himself to each soldier, leaving the stage with nothing left. When the tour was over, Lewis Black was exhausted and ready to head back home, but Robin got on a plane to Canada to film a movie. Lewis Black was incredulous, and said, "That was hard core. He's like a light that doesn't know how to turn itself off."

I have felt like that too: a little too much coffee, a few too many things on the to do list, and I could work all day, non-stop. But I am learning to reach for my own off switch and take the time to rest, and to visit the little altars in the day.

In Practice

Where can you create an altar in the day?
1. Start by finding one minute a day to close your eyes and focus on just breathing.
2. If at work, find a quiet room or sit in your car. If you have time, find a short guided meditation to listen to. Leslee Kagan, MS, FNP, has a fifteen minute "Body Scan Medition" on Spotify that I love.
3. Spend time in nature.
4. Sit and do nothing.
5. Read a page of something uplifting.
6. The 5-4-3-2-1 Method is a grounding exercise designed to manage acute stress and reduce anxiety. Name 5 things you can see, 4 things you can touch, 3 things you can hear, 2 things you can smell, and 1 thing you can taste.

18. Good Morning, Beautiful

"With the new day comes new strength and new thoughts."

—Eleanor Roosevelt

This is all such a work in progress, and I would love to say that I wake to my alarm going off not with a beep but to the sound of massive applause starting the day with a standing ovation, followed by sipping warm lemon water, writing in my gratitude journal, and then a meditation and forest walk before my breakfast of wheat grass juice and sun salutations.

BC (before cancer), I would jolt up, check Facebook and Instagram, take the dog out, and worry about the day ahead searching for missing socks.

I now aim for a happy medium and at least a sketch of a morning that will prime my nervous system for a calmer day.

I actually made a morning plan:

I want to wake up and put my hand on my chest and say a combination of a few things I've borrowed from different authors I love.

First, I wake up and start the day by saying, "Good morning, beautiful. I love you." Even if it feels cheesy.

Scarlet Keys

And then I say a little prayer:

Thank you God for perfect health, perfect healing, perfect harmony, and perfect homeostasis.

I imagine a white bubble of protection around the people I love.

Then I ask a question: "What wonderful thing could happen today?"

Then I say, "Today is going to be a great day, and everything always works out for me."

Then, I make my bed.

I have lemon water (not from a melted glacier, but filtered), and I look at a picture of myself when I was between six and ten, and I take a moment to love her. Or I look in the mirror and say, "I love you."

I meditate for at least five minutes, but ideally twenty. Sometimes, it's transcendental meditation, sometimes it's guided, but I love to set an intention for the day to be a patient and calm mom, a good partner, and helpful to my students, and mindful of my energy levels.

I make a plan—no matter how short—to have some kind of fun and leisure time that day.

I put on a song that makes me want to dance, and sometimes, I dance.

I exercise.

And then some days, I roll out of bed late and scramble to the car. It's practice, not perfection.

What If It All Goes Right?

> **In Practice**
>
> - How do you start your day?
> - How do you prime your nervous system?
> - How could you start your day in the best way to set yourself up for a calm and peaceful or productive day of work or leisure?
> - Set your alarm to the sound of applause so you start your day to a standing ovation? Or a song that lights you up?

19. The Alchemy of Gratitude

> *"Be grateful for your life, every detail of it, and your face will come to shine like the sun, and everyone who sees it will be made glad and peaceful. Persist in gratitude, and you will slowly become one with the sun of love, and love will shine through you its all-healing joy."*
>
> —Rumi

Just the *word* "Gratitude" can elicit an eye roll. When some well-meaning friend says "count your blessings," in impossible moments, it can feel more like they are tossing you a pint of ice-cream to smear on an open wound. It can be annoying and irritating when someone intercepts our feelings with a platitude when we are angry, scared, putting out a blazing fire, or on the edge of erupting into tears.

Phrases like "count your blessings" or "be grateful" have a bad rap and can feel trite and annoying, like a smiley face emoji, but there is a reason that things become clichés: it's because they work. Counting our blessings and being grateful is a spiritual practice that can be practiced any time, and there is now science to back up how expressing gratitude can benefit our health and our lives.

What If It All Goes Right?

Feeling gratitude can be a hard ask, and it can seem unachievable in certain situations. It's much easier to find gratitude in retrospect, after you're on the other side of adversity or heartbreak.

The thing about gratitude is that it is alchemistic. It changes our mental and emotional state suddenly.

One of the alchemistic features of gratitude is that we can't feel grateful and resentful, angry, annoyed, or scared at the same time. Gratitude is a lot like laughter, it takes over and changes things, like a red sock thrown into a load of white t-shirts.

Aside from acknowledging and honoring the real feelings that need to be named, felt, and expressed, I have found it crucial for my wellbeing for me to differentiate between feelings that *need* and *deserve* my attention and the undeserving and unnecessary feelings I inflict upon myself like dark rumination, nursing resentments, or imagining the worst.

Gratitude is available to us at any moment. Even sitting in the plastic dentist chair, white knuckling the armrest, we can begin: I am grateful I have insurance, I am grateful for the tree outside the window, or the ocean painting on the wall, and for this dentist who studied for years to save my tooth. I am grateful for the sweet dental assistant and for the music they have playing, and I'm grateful to have such good care.

We summon gratitude, and it rushes in like sunlight and floods the room. It will meet us where we are, from the courtroom to the hospital room, in a bend of a sun ray painting a strip of light on the white floor. Gratitude is here for us in all of its impossible magic.

One November, we drove to Maine to spend Thanksgiving with my mother-in-law. My cousin-in-law brought a big glass jar of cream with a few marbles in it. While we were waiting for dinner, we all sat in a circle in the living room and took turns shaking the jar. While we shook it, we would say what we were grateful for against the sounds of marbles ricocheting on the glass and then pass it to the next person. We went round and round until the cream turned to butter. It took about thirty minutes and when we were done, the room felt like it was filled with champagne bubbles. We sat down for dinner and spread our gratitude butter on our rolls and potatoes, and it brought the most wonderful feeling to the room.

Making gratitude a habit, such as starting the day with three different things you are grateful for, primes your day with positivity and sets your mental search engine to look for things to be grateful for. Savoring each thing on the list for a moment—bringing in the sensory experience of it—takes it a bit deeper, and ending each day with three things we are grateful for takes gratitude into sleep with us.

What we focus on expands, and in the words of Wayne Dyer, "When we change the way we look at things, the things we look at change." When we start to notice things about people in our lives that annoy us, *that* becomes the focus and only re-enforces the negative feelings that come with it. Everyone has faults and idiosyncrasies.

Instead of focusing on the loud volume of your partner's chewing and their facial skeletal acoustical abilities, and wondering if they shop for groceries by sound—like celery and pretzels—turn your attention to all the things you love about them. For an entire day, instead of focusing on their preternatural ability, focus on their laugh, how they care, how good it feels to sit next to them and feel calm and safe. It's kind of a partner half-empty/partner half-full situation, but it applies to everything.

We can brace ourselves for the day ahead by thinking about the worst parts of someone or the worst part of work, or we can be grateful and think about how we can be of service to others, make a difference, and the things we love about the people we love.

Gratitude Blast

When you really want to change the day, you can take a gratitude and appreciation challenge where you practice having gratitude for everything you see and experience. You do a gratitude blast for an entire hour. Remember that everything you have was once everything you wanted, so take stock. Stop and look around at all the things you wanted that you now have: I am grateful for this house, and this comfortable bed, and this big comfy pillow, and my sweet cat, and my dog, and my new floors, and my health, and my beating heart, and my car that's paid for, and the new paint on the walls, and that soft pink sweater. You can broaden that out to friends, work, neighbors, etc. That's all, total focus on everything you are grateful for.

Gratitude Day

To really throw glitter on the day, practice gratitude for the entire day. Focus on everything you love about your partner, your child, your job, your neighbor. Thank everything, every red traffic light that keeps you safe, the water flowing from your tap, the light that magically turns on because you flipped a switch, the hot shower, the internet, oh wow, a cell phone? amazing! on and on and on, and feel your moment, your body, your day change as you fill it up with appreciation.

Humorous Gratitude

If you don't like what you have, just think of all the things you don't want that you don't have. This can bring on a lot of laughter like, I'm so grateful I don't have a full body tattoo of Tony Danza I regret and now have to have removed.

Sometimes, when we have to do the boring adulty things, it's fun to think of things that would be worse to be doing. Like instead of complaining about your morning commute, you could be glad you're not going in on horse and buggy or waddling the entire 72 miles like the female penguin in *March of the Penguins* for just one fish.

What If It All Goes Right?

I had a friend who had been diagnosed with breast cancer and told me about how her husband Drew had bought a new jacket and spent the evening trying on different pants to match the jacket and asking several times if she was sure the jacket looked good on him. Then, one day when she was going in for radiation treatment, I sent her a text saying "Well, it could be worse. You could be cleaning out all of the port-a-potties in a small town, or extracting black heads from sumo wrestlers, or commenting on Drew's jacket one more time." She burst into laughter, and it made the day easier, and weirdly, brought a bit of gratitude through comparison and laughter. So, when you don't want to do something, make a list of ridiculous things you'd rather not do than the thing you have to do.

Retrospective Gratitude

Look back at pictures of great times you've had, and then make a gratitude list: I'm so grateful I got to see the Eiffel Tower, I'm so grateful for all the times my best friend made me laugh until I peed. I'm so grateful for that one day with my mom. I'm so grateful….

Anticipatory Gratitude

When we anticipate something we are looking forward to, there's an excitement to it. Positive anticipation releases the feel-good hormone dopamine. So, I'm so grateful for the vacation I'm going on, or the new music that's coming out, or getting to see my daughter in her new play, or reaching a milestone.

In Practice

Set a timer for ten minutes. Write without rhyme or rhythm, engaging as many of your senses as you can writing about what you are grateful for. "Show" don't "Tell," to really engage deeply and viscerally into your senses. Get detailed, writing about how the ceramic cup feels warm in your hand or how the swirl of steam rising up warms your face. The soft feel of your dog's white velvety ears or the sound and feel of the fall wind. I am so grateful for this bowl of pumpkin soup, and this rainy moment, and sitting next to my daughter, and the music that is playing in the background.

Engage all of your senses, bringing them in. Savor, relish, and bask in each one.

20. Laughter

"Laughter is the sun that drives winter from the human face."

—Victor Hugo

Laughter doesn't need a happy day. A good laugh is completely independent of circumstances and comes on like lightening in a black sky. Crackling across the night, lighting up the dark. Sometimes, it begins as a little giggle and escalates to a firework frenzy of body-shaking glee. It thrives on the absurd, ridiculous, inappropriate, and unexpected. I live for the kind of out-of-control laughing that leaves me folded over, red-faced, and even snorting. If I could bottle it, I would. It's a bit like a muse and a gift from the Gods, and it's an alchemist. It changes everything in an instant like turning on a light

David Lee wrote about laughter, "There's a certain kind of laughter that is a wildfire of contagious disaster. It's something that can't be anticipated or controlled."

The study of laughter is called "gelotology," from the Greek *gelos*, meaning "laughter." It explores how laughter effects the body from a psychological and physiological perspective, and focuses on the induction of laughter and its therapeutic effects in alternative medicine.

The scientific benefits of laughter include bringing in oxygenated air, activating our parasympathetic nervous system (provoking a calming effect). It boosts the immune system and floods the body with feel-good hormones, like dopamine, serotonin, and endorphins. It decreases adrenalin and cortisol. It is even known to lower blood pressure.

There is a lot of science that supports the therapeutic effects of laughing. Not fake party laughs, but *real* deep laughter. Dr. Norman Cousins famously used laughter as part of his healing a debilitating disease by watching funny movies over and over again.

Neuroimmunologists are scientists who study the interaction between our nervous and immune systems and have found that laughter helps us get rid of stress faster.

Even simulated laughter can be as effective as spontaneous laughter. They found that simulated laughter was even more effective at reducing depression and anxiety compared to spontaneous laughter. They recommend laughing sessions of at least three minutes, twice a week or more, for a minimum of six to eight weeks.

Simulated laughter feels silly and starts with a fake laugh, which you can try to turn into laughter that gradually becomes longer and louder. They say you can begin with using "ha-ha-ha" or "ho-ho-ho." You could try laughing like Chandler Bing's

What If It All Goes Right?

obnoxious girlfriend Janice from *Friends*. Just the absurdity can get you laughing. Experts recommend building up to three minutes of laughing. Instead of flooding our body with fear or dread, we are flooding it with good cheer and glee.

There is nothing more instantly transformative than laughter. Take a sad moment, an angry moment, an irritated moment, a scary moment; find the funny, and you instantly change your state of being. Laughter trumps all of these emotions, you can't be angry, sad, or scared and laugh at the same time.

Laughter isn't dependent on appropriate circumstances, and in fact, thrives in inappropriate and unexpected moments especially when it's discouraged and suppressed. Think of a kid bursting into flames of laughter in a church pew or the back of a classroom. It happens in work meetings and even sitting next to a funny irreverent friend at a funeral.

I think laughter is my favorite thing, and it has turned many heated moments into something sparkly and wonderful instead of serious and tense. I like to find the funny in the moment, and it feels so much better to laugh than to take things too seriously or to fight. I don't know why, but for me, talking in accents has really helped me survive things like my daughter's teen years. We both find the funny in a tense moment. Instead of a sharp tone, I will shift into saying what I need to say in the voice of a valley girl. It makes us both laugh and breaks the tension.

Sometimes, I lean on things that I know will make me laugh.

Scarlet Keys

In ACT (acceptance and commitment therapy), where something is scary, stressful or bothersome, we can defuse it by finding the funny in it. To complain, but complain with a German accent—for example, to lighten the moment. Suddenly, the phrase "My rotator cuff is not rotating" is funny. Another great technique is to sing the scary or stressful thing to a silly melody you know or make up. When you sing your fear to the tune of Barry Manilow's song "Copacabana," or to the tune of "Baby Shark," the hard feelings are diffused. It takes the sting out of it and usually brings on a little laughter.

Since we can't predict the lightning strike of laughter, and it's hard to force, I have found things that make me laugh.

My friend was visiting me from Australia and took me to a chemo appointment. She was sitting on the round stool the doctor usually sits on, with little rolling wheels. I said "Can you do something to make me laugh?" She said "I'm not funny," and I said, "Okay, I'll pull up a song on Spotify and you can dance." I put on a Nicki Minaj song called "Feeling myself" without ever hearing it before and had no idea what the lyrics were about. My sweet friend started dancing to that song with lyrics not written for infusion centers, and needless to say, I was in hysterics. I know the nurses outside the door were wondering how in the world I was laughing during treatments, but I also know they appreciated it.

If you can harness laughter in a stressful moment, you really do your body a favor, flooding it with feel-good hormones as your cortisol levels decrease.

What If It All Goes Right?

Another thing I do for stress release and finding laughter is asking my husband do the Argentine tango with me. Now this is an art form that takes years to master, so of course, I put the music on and we do what we call bad tango dancing through the house. It's so bad, we have no idea what we are doing, and the fact that my daughter can't stand it when we do this makes us laugh even harder. We even grab a leaf off a plant or a flower for our teeth and usually fall over in complete laughter at how bad we are.

I take advantage of the fact that my husband is so funny and has a gift for physical comedy. When nothing is funny and laughter isn't happening organically, I try to find it and create it.

I have what I call my "laughing friends"—the people I know I can call and end up laughing with every time. They are a treasure to me, and I literally will call them and say I need to laugh today.

Anything unexpectedly silly often brings on at least a chuckle or a smile. I might put on a tiara while folding laundry and see how long it takes my husband to notice, and that makes me laugh. My best friend of over thirty years, always makes me laugh. She will stop at nothing for a laugh and I can't remember a time we've spent over all these years where we didn't fall over howling.

I look for the ridiculous and ironic things in life and try to actively find the funny.

So many journal practices start and end each day asking you to think about three things that you are grateful for. We start to find what we look for. So, try adding a funny search. At the end of each day, ask "What made me laugh today?" Maybe it didn't make it to laughing status, and there was no snorting or crying laughter, but maybe even a chuckle or a snicker? It begins to put funny on the map for your life.

What If It All Goes Right?

In Practice

Here are a few things to help you light the match of funny:
1. Spend time with people who make you laugh.
2. Watch or listen to stand-up comics.
3. Watch funny videos or movies, or read a funny book.
4. Diffuse difficult emotions and situations by complaining in a humorous accent.
5. Buy something silly for your family, like Slinkies at the dinner table.
6. Do something big and fun, like go to Harry Potter World.
7. End each day with the question, "What made me laugh today?"

21. Friendship

"When friendships are real, they are not glass threads or frost work, but the solidest things we can know."

—Ralph Waldo Emerson

Friendship is a hand on your shoulder, and sometimes, its two hands folded in prayer. Friendship is an out of the blue soul quake of laughter that only the laughing understand. It is a wide, whole-hearted hug. It is an angel's breath on the back of your neck whispering, "Yes, you can." It fiercely keeps your secrets in the vault and stands loyal and tall. Friendship is an altar where you lay down your truth and your broken parts and says, "I love you, or "Me too."

Friendship finds you where you are but doesn't leave you where it found you, it takes your hand and sets you down on higher ground. It holds up a mirror but sees you in the perfect light. It lets you "ugly cry" and says "no" when you ask if your life makes you look fat. It reminds you of your dream and talks you out of quitting. It cheers you on from the sidelines and the bleachers and is there at the finish line with a smile that feels like it belongs to you. It brings up your name in a room full of opportunity and throws confetti when you win. It weighs its words before it

What If It All Goes Right?

speaks and is called to forgive again and again. It says what it means, but it doesn't say it mean. It struggles with jealousy but finds a way to be happy for you when you get the thing they most wanted because it feels like it's happening for them too.

Friendship says the hard thing like "Are you sure you want that glass of wine?" and also knows the power of silence. It reminds us who we truly are, and we like ourselves best when we are with them. When it walks in the door, our heart doesn't brace itself; it sparkles like champagne, open-armed. It admits when it is wrong and can't stand one day of being mad at you and will drive across town to make things right. It fights *with* you and *for* you.

A friend is a rare treasure that holds your hand and doesn't ask what they can do. It just shows up at the door with the casserole and flowers.

We need people. We need community and confidants. We need to be understood and to feel connected. No man is an island.

Loneliness has such far-reaching consequences that the health impact is comparable to smoking up to fifteen cigarettes a day, according to one study published in the journal *PLOS Medicine*.

Loneliness is associated with an increased risk of heart disease, depression, and cognitive decline.

We need each other to thrive and to be happy and well.

When I was going through treatment, I needed my friends. In person, on the phone, in texts, and virtually. I had to learn to receive help. It felt awkward and powerless being checked in on and coddled, but my friends and my community literally held me up when I couldn't hold myself.

I love being the one who brings the casserole and is there for my friends, but I was just too depleted and overwhelmed.

I didn't have anything to give, and it was really a struggle to be looked in on and taken care of by the people I love. But it was really the most wonderful and life-affirming thing to know how much people care. There is healing in just knowing that we matter to people. It's a hard gift, but it's a gift to find out just how much people care about you and love you. It's a beautiful thing to know.

Just getting a card in the mail or a phone call or a text or email with someone checking in can buoy us on a difficult day.

Having connections with neighbors and friends, workmates, and family is vital.

Our longevity is deeply affected by the quality of our relationships. It's not just about how many people we know or call "friend" but the *quality* of those interactions. I try to spend time with people who leave me better than they found me—who make me laugh or learn and leave me feeling energized and not depleted or deflated. I pay attention to the energy of the people around me and try to hold those sparkly souls close.

How often are you in touch with your closest friends or family? How could you make time to

What If It All Goes Right?

strengthen your connection to them? It's important to maintain and strenghten our friendships.

When something reminds me of a friend, just writing them a note saying "This reminded me of you" or "I thought you might like this" is a nice way to connect. I also love when I come across an old photo of a good time we had together, I send it to them out of the blue.

In a society where productivity and product are king, we have to make a conscious effort to stay connected. As Emerson said, "The only way to have a friend is to be one."

In Practice

1. Text two people you haven't been in touch with in a while. It can be as simple as "Hello!" or "Thinking of you today."
2. Hold a Zoom party. Invite people you've missed who live far away.
3. Schedule a get-away with your favorite people.
4. Invite a friend over for coffee.
5. Reach out to someone interesting with whom you would like to build a friendship.
6. Ask for help and offer help.

Ways to Make New Friends

1. Join a new group dedicated to something you've always wanted to try.
2. Look to your local library for group activities.
3. Join a place of worship.
4. Volunteer.
5. Take a class.
6. "Friend" new people on Facebook in your community, and comment on their posts. I made one of my best friends from Facebook and commenting on her artwork.
7. Join a cause, like a walk for a cause.
8. Take a self-help seminar.
9. Go back to school.
10. Get a dog, and meet new people in your neighborhood.

22. A Good Cry

> *"There is a sacredness in tears. Tey are not the mark of weakness, but of power. They speak more eloquently than ten thousand tongues. They are the messengers of overwhelming grief, of deep contrition, and of unspeakable love."*
>
> —Washington Irving

Ugly cry, angry cry, lonely cry, grief cry, joy cry, religious cry it doesn't matter why, just cry. Any cry is a good cry.

There are some days when we don't want to make a gratitude list or hunt down joy, or force a laugh. Some days we just need to cry.

In a philosophy class I took in college, my professor had the class make a list of the saddest movies we had ever seen. Movies that made us cry. And he said that it didn't matter why we cried, as long as we cried. Even releasing tears in response to something other than what is currently upsetting us can be healthy.

When we hold things in and don't allow space for our emotions, they can build and leak out at weird times—often disguised as more acceptable emotions like anger or indignation, or "justified" road rage.

Scarlet Keys

Crying is important for our emotional wellbeing. But crying is uncomfortable, and rare, for some of us. I need the right setting, and it often requires solitude unless something weird triggers it like arriving at the parking garage with ten minutes to spare before I teach a class to hear the attendant yell, "The lot if full, there's no space!" I drive away in tears like he had just yelled, "You are worthless, and your car makes you look fat."

Crying in front of other people is such a vulnerable act and is sometimes associated with embarrassment and even shame. Women often apologize when they cry. Wiping back tears, saying "I'm sorry."

So many men indoctrinated in toxic masculinity are made fun of and told to man up. And none of us want to be seen as weak and crying at work of all places. All this has done is led to a culture damned up with tears with no outlet—a river with nowhere to go.

Crying can be hard because of the busyness of our culture. We don't give it time. Who has time to cry?

Tears aren't only a response to cutting onions or fighting against irritants. They are there to release feelings of sadness, anguish, loneliness, and stress.

We are meant to cry. That's why we have tear ducts.

What If It All Goes Right?

There are three types of tears:
- Basal tears: Lubricate, nourish, and protect our eyes.
- Reflex tears: Wash away irritants. Basal and reflex tears contain salt, fatty oils, and over 1,500 different proteins.
- Emotional tears: Contain natural pain killers and stress hormones.

According to Harvard Health, researchers note that, on average, American women cry 3.5 times each month, while American men cry about 1.9 times each month. Crying is good for us and allows us to release stress and emotional pain. Stuffing our feelings or being too busy to feel them suppresses our immune system and affects our cardiovascular and mental health negatively.

Researchers know that crying releases oxytocin and endorphins. But we can't heal what we won't feel, and we often need to take the time to get in touch with how we feel.

Photographer Rose-Lynn Fisher spent a decade magnifying and photographing her tears, learning the nuances of her emotions in the process.

The Topography of Tears is a visual investigation of tears that she photographed through an optical standard light microscope. Fisher wondered what tears look like and saved her tears on glass slides. The pictures she took were astonishing, and each type of tear had a different pattern.

Scarlet Keys

Tears have different shapes, patterns, and chemical makeup depending on why you are crying.

Each tear has its own chemical makup, much like a snowflake.

While I was still having chemotherapy, I had lovely, well-meaning neighbors reach out in texts or emails saying, "If you ever just need to call someone and let it all out, I'm here." I appreciated that, but to really be able to let it go, I had to be with someone I felt at home with. My best friend from high school and I had reconnected after many years, and she made that same offer to me one day. I tucked that sweet offer away, and then weeks later, I had to go to the grocery store and had forgotten my wig. I was with my teenage daughter and had just heard about someone having a recurrence and becoming terminal, and just the day before, someone called me sir at the post office. I was feeling vulnerable, and exposed, in a store with total strangers looking at my bald head.

I have always had long thick curly hair and this was really hard. When I got home, my husband and daughter went to the beach, and I called my friend and I cried for half an hour. I felt so much better. It was a good cry.

I felt like I had an emotional reset and that I could face the next thing.

Having a safe place to cry and a genuine listener is a rare and wonderful thing.

What If It All Goes Right?

In Practice

How often do you cry? What helps you access the feelings that would be helped by a good cry?

Try making time for your feelings.

1. Write. Write it all down, knowing that no one will read what you write and then burn it, throw it away, or keep it. I love the E.M. Forster quote, "How do I know what I think until I see what I say?"
2. Watch a really sad movie alone or with someone else who is as sappy as you are, and let it all out.
3. Take a long drive, and let it all out.
4. Listen to music that can get you in touch with your sadness.
5. Sit with a good friend who you can cry with.

23. What's Your Soundtrack?

"Beautiful music is the art of the prophets that can calm the agitations of the soul. It is one of the most magnificent and delightful presents God has given us."

—Martin Luther

We all listen to and turn to music. Songs are the soundtracks of our lives. Think of the events of your life, and chances are, there is a song you can connect to a season or a moment. From lullabies to birthday parties, camp songs, church hymns, your first kiss, your wedding song, your next wedding song, your breakup song, your fight song, and songs played at funerals. The right song amplifies our experiences in the same way a great film score affects a movie.

The right song can make hard things less hard, make us hate sitting in traffic a little less, make us dance, let us cry, help us run the extra mile, and face scary things with more bravery. A song is both a time capsule and a time machine. Songs hold moments for us and help us remember our lives.

When we listen to music we love, our body releases the feel-good hormone dopamine. When we listen to music we don't like, our bodies release the stress hormone cortisol. Think about how waiting on

What If It All Goes Right?

the phone with terrible hold music makes you feel. Or the way you feel when your favorite song comes on out of nowhere.

Listening to certain music can lower our blood pressure. A song can change the weather in the room and change how we feel.

When our kids wake up grumpy or late and stressed, the morning becomes a house of different moods. The quickest way I've found to change the emotional atmosphere of my house on such a morning, and to unify a room, is to put on a song I know everyone will love. Without my saying a word, we're all in sync to the same tempo and groove of the song that is playing, and the music helps move the morning into a better space. Now, instead of launching into the day with stress or a fight over who ate the last bit of cereal, we are all dancing out the door to the groove of "Happy" by Pharrell. Try this when you have challenging visitors, too. Put on a song you know they will like, and let the dopamine flow and unite the room in a way that only music can.

There were so many days on the way to a treatment that I prepared a playlist for the car and a playlist for while I was actually in treatment. My favorite music flooded the moment and filled the air, calming my nervous system, and making me feel stronger.

As someone who writes songs and who mentors other songwriters, I can take this readily available tool—music—for granted. But during my hardest time, I went back to being an audience and back to the person I once was who leaned on a good song to get me through.

This year, one of my playlist songs was Lizzo's "About Damn Time." It was the summer jam for thousands of her fans. For me, it was my fight song while going through treatment for breast cancer.

This song felt like it was written just for me and the song's groove and lyrics got me through by changing my body's chemistry and lightening me up emotionally with a message I really needed to hear.

What is your fight song? Your feel-good song? Your traffic jam song? Your wake-up or dancing-in-the-shower song? Your breakup song? Your find-love-again song?

We can curate the soundtrack of our lives. What song could you play instead of dwelling on something worrisome? What song do you want to hear when you start your day? Dance in the shower to? What is the fight song you could blast before before you walk into an important meeting or when you need to feel stronger? A great morning song can do so much to prime our nervous systems for a better day and is a great way to bypass any automatic negative thoughts.

Songs can help us tackle boring and dreaded tasks, such as doing our taxes, paying bills, doing laundry, and vacuuming. Since my focus has been on avoiding unnecessary low-vibration feeling states such as dread and boredom, putting on music that I love or that makes me dance or move can make these tasks less torturous.

What If It All Goes Right?

Try the following:
- The next time you clean the kitchen or do the dishes, put on Latin music and dance while you do it.
- Vacuum to your guilty-pleasure pop song.
- Exercise to songs that make you feel amazing.

Songs can activate the life-changing emotions of wonder and awe. Think of great classical music or gospel songs. When we sing with others, our body releases the love hormone oxytocin.

Songs can also diffuse negative emotions. Try taking something that is stressful, like the guy who cut you off in traffic, and sing about it to the tune of "Like a Virgin." You will defuse the stress and hopefully even laugh.

As I've gotten older, I've been horrified by some of the nouns I've had to add to my vocabulary, such as *jowls* and *turkey neck*. Most recently, I was accused of being eligible for a senior discount and then heard about how women's skin texture changes as their hormones change and was then introduced to the term "crepey skin." I was so upset that I did the only thing a songwriter could do, and I wrote a song.

"Crepe Skin"

Verse 1

Getting' old's no joke when you used to be smokin' hot
Startin' fires with your crotch
Turnin' heads, burnin' beds,
then it stops, hormones drop, then you've got
Crepe skin
When you go to take a selfie, hold the cell phone higher
Tilt your head try to find a better light
There's no denyin' and there's no escapin'
Crepe skin

Chorus:

Crepe skin, oh I got
Crepe skin

V2. *I'm just getting' started,*
Haven't figured out the journey yet
Better than I've ever been, but now I have a turkey neck
So I start wearing scarfs like Diane Keaton
Turtle-neck sweaters in the summer when it's heatin'

(Chorus)

V3. *Silver is the new blonde*
Puttin' the stilettos on
I'm gonna play the Fender
swipe to the right on Tinder

What If It All Goes Right?

I walk into a room, I'm there for the party
And I'm a member of the AARP
Age is just a number, still got the thunder,
I ain't goin' under
With my skin tags, leg cramps, hot flash, mammograms
Dizzy and forgettin' sweatin' frettin' with eye bags

(Chorus)

V4. *I won't give in to the fillers or the Botox*
I'm gonna spread some shimmer
and some glitter on my age spots
I still got it, I blot it, I flaunt it, I blonde it,
I rock it, I gloss it, I'm on it, salon it, applaud it,
I'm on it, I'm on it
I prop it wearin' long sleeves
with my bat wings elephant knees
Thinning hair and lost keys
And frequent urination

(Chorus)

V5. *The audacity of gravity*
randomly attacking my anatomy, this alchemy
Got me misshapin' and grayin',
weighin' savin' what's remainin',
But I can't escape the changin'
or erase the accelerated agin'
But I've got crepatitude a new attitude
I'm wider but wiser and finer in my designer diaper
And I love, I love, I love
My crepe skin

Songs are great therapy. Dr. Dan Siegel developed a strategy for parents to use in the midst of big emotions called "Name It to Tame It" to help children name their overwhelming emotions through words. Songs also do that for us. They put a name to what we are feeling, and lyrics help us label our emotions. These words are amplified by the music and can help us express and resolve emotions and feel understood and less alone.

In Practice

1. Create a playlist of songs that support a feeling you want to express or experience. It coudl be sadness, strenght, hope, anger, bravery, love, etc.
2. Write a song.

Here are some of the songs from my playlists. What playlists can you create for yourself?

Morning Songs
- "Lovely Day" Bill Withers
- "I Smile" Kirk Franklin
- "Happy" Pharrell Williams
- "Let Your Love Flow" the Bellamy Brothers
- "Walk with Me" GoldFord
- "Best Day of My Life" American Authors

What If It All Goes Right?

Songs for Strength
- "Brave" Don Diablo with Jessie J
- "Rise Up" Andra Day
- "Stand Up" Cynthia Erivo
- "A Million Dreams" Pink
- "Fight Song" Rachel Platten
- "Broken & Beautiful" Kelly Clarkson
- "Fighter" Christina Aguilera
- "You Got It Girl" Drake & Chris Brown

Feel-Good Songs
- "Hold On (Change Is Comin')" Sounds of Blackness
- "Higher Love" Whitney Houston
- "Beautiful Day" U2
- "I Can See Clearly Now" Johnny Nash
- "O-o-h Child" Roberta Flack
- "Joyful, Joyful" Pentatonix, Jazmine Sullivan
- "My Revival" Morgxn
- "Love Is the Answer" England Dan & John Ford Coley
- "So You" Coma Estereo
- "Don't You Worry 'bout a Thing" Stevie Wonder
- "Up" Tauren Wells
- "Somehow, Someway" Chad Price
- "Crown" Chika
- "Diamonds" Johnnyswim
- "Praise" Lady Bri
- "No Bad Days" Macklemore feat. Collett

24. Awe and Wonder

"But if a man be alone, let him look at the stars. The rays that come from those heavenly worlds, will separate between him and vulgar things. One might think the atmosphere was made transparent with this design, to give man, in the heavenly bodies, the perpetual presence of the sublime. Seen in the streets of cities, how great they are! If the stars should appear one night in a thousand years, how would men believe and adore; and preserve for many generations the remembrance of the city of God which had been shown! But every night come out these envoys of beauty, and light the universe with their admonishing smile."

—Ralph Waldo Emerson

Awe is defined as a feeling of reverential respect mixed with fear or wonder.

When we focus on the wondrous, we elevate the moment and transcend the way we feel. When we are full of wonder or awe, there's no room for any other feeling.

Even in the most difficult moment, we can access wonder and turn our attention to the sacred or something that elicits reverence.

What If It All Goes Right?

Even on the hardest day, we can step outside and just look up at the sky, the treetops, the early morning sunlight, or notice geese flying in formation. If we're lucky, maybe there is a rainbow after the rain.

When awe and wonder feel out of reach, I can recall a memory of awe, like taking a helicopter ride inside a dormant volcano in Kauai and seeing a waterfall. My eyes filled with tears to see that kind of untouched beauty. I recall a time seeing the ocean light up with phosphoresce dragging my fingers through the water at night on a sailboat and the four-hour fondue dinner in a small restaurant tucked in the side of a mountain in Austria. Then, I can think of the time I got to stand on stage with Carly Simon and sing "Lean on Me" at the end of a concert I had been a part of on Martha's Vineyard, years ago. I know I was only standing there because I was part of the show, but I was literally basking in those unforgettable three and a half minutes.

When it comes to high quality emotions, "Awe" is in a category all to itself.

It is one of the top emotions that puts our body in a high feeling state.

When we experience awe, it puts things in perspective.

What do you associate with the following words:

AHHH   *ah-a*   *awesome*   *awed*   *amen*

Awe is a part of all these words.

Of course, there is *awful*, where we are stunned by something horrific like a hurricane or bad behavior, but for the purposes of this chapter, we will focus on the positive effects of Awe and the sense of wellbeing it can offer.

There is wide-lens awe, the Northern Lights, and an astronaut's view as she leaves gravity, staring back weightlessly at our great blue planet. There is seeing your child being born or meeting the pope or Dalai Lama, or seeing Taylor Swift in a sea of Swifties at her concert.

Then there are everyday moments of awe, like noticing the birch tree in the parking lot of the doctor's office with its fall leaves gold against the white trunk. Waiting in the office, you could look out the window and find something small to spark even the tiniest flicker of awe, like the morning light in the sky, or on a cold winter day, apricity (the warmth of sun in the winter). It can always be found in the sky and in nature, and we can actively seek it out.

Heroic acts, generosity, and kindness elicit awe in the people who witness it. This is called "moral beauty."

I had a student years ago who had been a soldier in Afghanistan. When he returned from duty, he decided to pursue his dream and attend Berklee. His songs always tackled important topics, and I could see how much he cared about humanity in the songs he wrote that were geared towards social change.

What If It All Goes Right?

He was married and had a small child, and one day he was reading the paper and came across an article about a young woman who had given her father a kidney, but it had recently failed so she was asking for a donor. He thought "what if I'm the only match and could save his life?" So, he reached out, got tested, and it turned out, he was a match. He met the family, and shortly after, was in the hospital giving a total stranger a kidney. Everyone who knew him was amazed and inspired, as he was zooming in to classes from his hospital bed as he recovered, not missing an assignment. We were all moved and touched by this huge act of generosity. It's the kind of act you never forget.

About a year later, I ran into him, and he was despondent. I asked what was wrong, and he said, the kidney failed, it was all for nothing. But he wasn't mourning the loss of his kidney, he was morning the loss of the life of the stranger he had come to know. I said "It wasn't for nothing, you have inspired everyone who knows you and has heard about this story, and that is not nothing."

Everyone involved is still impacted all these years later.

I am always in awe when someone tells the truth, especially the hard embarrassing truth, and it always gives the people listening permission to tell their truth.

It inspired awe when Taylor Swift was changing the economy with her Era's tour, reading about how she wrote each one of her truck drivers a check for $100,000 dollars with a handwritten note made everyone love her even more.

When we hear about anonymous giving, it has even more impact.

Dr. Declan Keltner is a professor at UC Berkeley, and his research shows that awe "is its own thing," and says that our bodies respond differently when we are experiencing awe than when we are feeling joy, contentment, or fear. We make a different sound, show a different facial expression. He defines awe as a sense of wonder, an experience of mystery, that transcends our understanding. These, it turns out, are as common in human life globally as they are measurably health-giving and immunity-boosting. They bring us together with others, again and again. They bring our nervous system and heartbeat and breath into sync—and even into sync with other bodies around us.

It also has psychological benefits. Many of us have a critical voice in our head, telling us we're not smart, handsome, or rich enough. Awe seems to quiet this negative self-talk by deactivating the default mode network—the part of the cortex involved in how we perceive ourselves.

Instead of asking my daughter to play the license plate game when we are driving, I will ask her to look out the window and find something awesome. When we look for wonder, we add that search engine to our

What If It All Goes Right?

brain, and we start to find it. We also begin to feel the effects of this emotion. Instead of asking our child how their day was, we could ask them "What was amazing today?"

In Practice

Exercises in awe:

1. Look for awe and wonder throughout your day.
2. At the end of each day, write down one thing that made you feel a sense of awe.
3. Commuting to work, you could notice the sky, or the fall trees lining the highway.
4. Read a book or watch a movie about an inspiring figure.
5. Read quotes from a writer who inspires awe.
6. Look at pictures of things that inspire awe in you.
7. Watch Carl Sagan's video *The Pale Blue Dot*."
8. Go on an awe walk, and notice the miraculous from a squirrels nest to a bird taking a dirt bath.
9. Spend time in nature.
10. Close your eyes and recall three moments of awe or wonder.

25. Woo-Woo

"I believe in mystery and, frankly, I sometimes face this mystery with great fear. In other words, I think that there are many things in the universe that we cannot perceive or penetrate, and that also we experience some of the most beautiful things in life only in a very primitive form. Only in relation to these mysteries do I consider myself to be a religious man…"

—Albert Einstein

Woo-woo is considered to be connected with paranormal and pseudoscientific phenomena. And it's usually used in a derogatory way. But there are things that fall under this category that have benefited me.

I have been calling this year my Year of Woo. I haven't gone full woo, just woo-ish.

I remember working at a restaurant in San Diego with a manager, who was completely stressed and probably coked out. There was a head waitress there who had just been deeply introduced to all things new age, and one day, the manager was in a rage and standing at a cash register about to explode. The head waitress stood behind him doing a ritual, and he yelled, "STOP FLUFFING MY AURA!" It was one of the funniest things I've ever seen.

Scarlet Keys

I never give any thought to horoscopes or what the new moon might mean or blaming my lost keys on Mercury being in retrograde. I don't care about any of my past lives, as I'm just trying to get through this one.

But my Year of Woo has included things like Reiki, healing crystals, believing in better and higher angels, and staying open to anything that might be healing or beneficial. Including fluffing an aura or two.

So far, I have said yes to Reiki, crystals, affirmations, burning sage, sound healing, wearing essential oils, and to a spiritual weekend retreat where upon arrival, the leader swirled a pot of white billowing sage while cleansing my energy. I thought, "I guess we're doing this," but I honestly felt a little better. Then, we walked up to the top of a hill with fall leaves dancing all around us, surrounded by huge sculptures, as we did a heart meditation. We then walked up to an even more enormous open field and had a cocoa and rose drink ceremony to heal our hearts as the woman leading the event did a meditation. She asked us why we were there, and when I introduced myself and talked about my health year, she said, "You have been challenged to come back to yourself." That felt true to me.

She talked about chakras and the cosmos and other things I couldn't digest, as I just watched the clouds float above the dancing leaves. We then went back to a lodge, and she taught us the ancient Hawaiian practice that combines love, forgiveness, repentance, and gratitude, in four powerful phrases for any time you experience conflict.

What If It All Goes Right?

It's called Hoʻoponopono:
1. I'm sorry.
2. Please forgive me.
3. I thank you.
4. I love you.

There was a tray of crocheted little potatoes holding signs. I picked one at random and turned it over, and it said, "You are returning to yourself." That felt woo-woo but meant to be.

I am now in pursuit of my second woo, where I will be trying: liver cleanse, foot bath to remove toxins, meditation retreat, acupuncture and cupping, and spiritual workshops.

A great place to find things like this is on flyers at your local coffee shop. In fact, that's where I write, in coffee shops. On my last writing break, I took a picture of three different flyers. One was a meditation and movement class, one was a qigong class, and the other was a sound mediation class that read "Open, breathe, let go." I am going to try one in honor of woo.

What could you stay open-minded to? What Woo could you try for better health, wellness, fun, and adventure?

In Practice

Finding Woo:
- Look online for a woo you're curious about.
- Schedule a Reiki session or something woo that you could try.

26. What If It All Goes Right?

> *"Don't worry, You don't know enough to worry. That's God's truth. Who do you think you are that you should worry, for crying out loud? It's a total waste of time. It presupposes such a knowledge of the situation that it is in fact a form of hubris."*
>
> —Terence McKenna

I teach lyric writing, and in my class, I talk about the power of using interrogatives—that is, questions. Taylor Swift often uses interrogatives in her lyrics, and it's a great way to connect with your audience and involve them. Lyrics such as "Are you ready for it?" and "What's that like?" and "If the story's over, why am I still writing pages?" When we ask a question, it begs for an answer or a consideration. There is an energy in it.

Instead of declaring, predicting or preparing for the worst try asking a question: What if it all goes right? What wonderful thing could happen today? What beautiful thing could come from this? What amazingly kind people could I encounter today? It asks the universe to answer that question.

What If It All Goes Right?

If that's too far of a stretch, you could start with, "What if it doesn't all go wrong?" or "What if something unexpected and difficult arises, but I handle it with grace?"

It's true that not everything goes as planned. The things that *do* go wrong are rarely the things we worried about. They are things we couldn't have predicted, but we got through. We handled it, and the proof is that here we are on the other side of it.

If imagining the worst is just the misuse of imagination, let's go ahead and do our nervous systems a favor and use the power of imagination for good and expect a favorable outcome. If something unforeseen and difficult happens, we can handle it in the moment it belongs to and not all the moments leading up to the dreaded future happening.

Dread is a terrible emotion to steep ourselves in. It feels terrible. So does imagining the worst: it's like watching a horror movie over and over again. Why do that to ourselves?

When we expect something good, there is a sparkling feeling to it that feels good to our body. It feels good to our nervous systems, and that translates to our immune system and overall wellbeing.

There is a grace in all of us—a hidden strength that waits to be summoned. We are never alone, even in the hardest moment, and it feels good to have a little faith. If something hard or dark or even terrible happens, we will rise to the occasion like the super-strength the woman gets when she lifts a car off a child after an accident. We are so much more than our nervous imaginings: we are grit and grace with an inner resource that knows we were made to do hard things.

We can't predict anything, so in the meantime, while we are waiting for the test result, the phone call, the plane to land, the envelope to be opened, the storm to pass, what if…we ask the question "What if it all goes right?" Or at least "What if it all goes better than planned?" Or the very least, "What if it doesn't go horribly?"

It actually *could* go well, it *could* be that we get the best possible outcome, it could be that the whole world is conspiring *for* us!

Think about something right now you are worried about. Now take a moment to scan your body for tension. How do you breathe when you are worried? Are your muscles tense? Are your fists clenched? What about tightness in your jaw? Any adrenaline running through your veins?

Thoughts are powerful things, so now…ask yourself this question: How would you breathe if you knew everything was going to be okay? If everything was going to work out? How would you act if you were in perfect health? How would you walk if you knew the whole world loved you? Would your shoulders be relaxed? Would you breathe easy? Even smile?

Now, take a moment to stand or sit the way you would if you just received a divine announcement that you were just fine and everything was going to

What If It All Goes Right?

go well. Now, hold that feeling. Let yourself have this.

We have a choice on how we experience the moments leading up to an event. Yes, fearful imaginings are going to enter our minds and our hearts will race and our breathing will become shallow, but we can catch that moment of terror by being aware and mindful. When that worst-case scenario flashes in our mind, we can say "stop," and then breathe deeply, and let our bodies relax, and divert our attention and our day to something real and worthy of our time.

"What if it all goes right?"

When I had to have my chemo port removed, I asked a friend what it was like when she had hers taken out. In a very stressed tone, she went into detail about how terrible it was. That was hard to hear, and it worried me, but the day of my port removal, I decided to think, "What if all of my doctors and nurses are wonderful, and it all goes well?"

Walking into the hospital that morning, an elderly gentleman was walking out, and he made a really funny, unexpected joke to me and my husband that made us crack up. I walked in with that levity and had such a nice interaction with the front desk greeter, the nurse taking my blood, and the doctor in the surgery room prepping me. We even laughed. I did feel a little bit of pain when they numbed the chest area, but that was it. When they took the port out, I didn't even feel a thing or notice. They took me to the recovery room, and then they made me the best grilled-cheese sandwich I've ever had, with

Scarlet Keys

really good iced tea. Every nurse was wonderful, and it all went well. I handled a little bit of pain when they took blood and when they numbed me, but there was goodness all around me, and even the computer screen in my recovery room said "loving kindness" on the screen. That hospital is on "Loving Kindness Drive" in York, Maine.

So, let's dare to imagine the best, knowing we can handle anything that is unexpected. Expect the best, and enjoy our lives until a hard thing actually happens. Enjoy our one precious life, and let each day be full of as much happiness, fun, love and wonder as our nervous hearts can stand. Let's leave the dark days where they belong because maybe all of our dark days are behind us, and maybe—just maybe (as Frank Sinatra famously sang), "It's a real good bet, the best is yet to come."

What If It All Goes Right?

> **In Practice**
>
> Wake up each morning and ask yourself:
> - What wonderful thing could happen today?
> - What if everyone I meet is lovely and kind?
> - What if today will be lined with sunlight"
> - What if it all goes right?

27. New Management

"The world as we have created it is a process of our thinking. It cannot be changed without changing our thinking."

—Albert Einstein

The past few years have been me trying to turn the ocean liner of my life around and making changes in the way I live, to give my body a better environment for healing and wellness. I had someone say to me on more than one occasion, "You need new management," and we would laugh as I was called out for once again saying "yes" to something I didn't really want to do, or the time I left a paradise vacation early to drive three hours to meet an old friend who was visiting from out of town only to hear (after forty-five minutes at lunch), "Well, good to see you, we're gonna go back to our hotel."

If you could hire a manager to come in and assess the way you are living, what would they find? What would their report look like?

The first place I looked was at the things that caused stress in my life. But I had to differentiate between the everyday stress that life can bring and self-inflicted stress, and there is a huge difference.

What If It All Goes Right?

For a clear, non-biased opinion, it might be helpful to consult the people in your life who know you well or who live with you, if they can identify any actions, inactions, or things that they feel cause you unnecessary stress.

Organization

I lose my keys and my phone often, and in fact, there are several other things I lose, too. So, I made a list of all of the things I frantically search for while swearing. Any noun that used the adjective F*ing in front of it made the list.

Where are my:
- F*ing glasses
- F*ing keys
- F*ing scissors
- F*ing Scotch tape
- F*ing phone
- F*ing tweezers
- F*ing nail clippers
- F*ing wallet
- F*ing Band-Aids
- F*ing PHONE CHARGER

I know that some people reading this are killing the whole adulting thing, and alphabetize their underwear, but there are some of us who struggle with these seemingly simple things. When we are stressed, our executive functioning is often affected and not working well. Becoming more organized has simplified my life. And most importantly, it has alleviated some of the undue stress.

So… I did the obvious. I made a place for those F*ing things on my list and bought extra cables, scissors, and tweezers, etc., because I have other people in my home who use these things and then no one can find the F*ing anything!

I read somewhere that when we can't remember where we left something or where we parked in a parking garage, it's because we didn't take a moment to remember it. We can't remember something we don't observe, so I learned that when I put my glasses down or my keys, I have to take a moment to slow down and observe where I put them—or better yet, to put them in their assigned place. But frantically looking for things while saying the F word had to change!

Being Late

I've looked at my late habit. There is no use arriving late to a yoga class, speeding up on the curb like Cruella de Vil. I've even abandoned the "just in time" rebrand and decided to become an early person. Arriving early and waiting for the other people to arrive at the meeting allows me the rare pleasure and undeserved air of superiority. But seriously, I have alleviated transitional stress. I arrive really early, and then I can read, or mediate, or take a walk, or look at the world around me, or have a conversation with a workmate that's relaxed and present. No Rush!

Commuting

Leaving early makes driving a lot less stressful. I sometimes put a flower on my dashboard, and I no longer talk on the phone while driving. It's just

What If It All Goes Right?

asking too much of my body to have a conversation, listening while dodging cars, and trying not to die in traffic. I either listen to music or a podcast or an audio book. It is so much more soothing and relaxing then driving and talking. I take the bus when I really want to relax or get work done.

Thinking

Our thoughts are powerful, so I have definitely included taking stock in and being aware of the thoughts I choose and those that no longer serve me.

Procrastination

Then, there was the procrastination habit, and yes, there is a thrill and a surge of adrenaline that occurs with a deadline. But I've been turning my stress ocean-liner around and heading for smoother waters, so I also added doing things now or earlier than expected. This has taken so much stress out of my life. I have observed from the most organized people I know that they do things NOW. They drive up to their house, grab the mail, bring the trash can back in, and when they get in the door, they sort the mail NOW. When they cook, they clean as they go. Neat people follow the old:
- Don't pass it up, pick it up.
- Don't put it down, put it away.

Procrastination isn't a kind thing to do to our future selves. When we put things off, we are really just handing our future self hours of taxes to sort,

Scarlet Keys

hours of laundry to do, hours of stress, because it's a task handed to the future. "Do it NOW" is my new motto. Or "Do some of it NOW."

When we have had childhood trauma or a chaotic upbringing, we can be comfortable with chaos and drama. I hated to admit it but it's true: I was a bit of a cortisol junkie and thrived on adrenaline. I had to find a mantra and practice for getting comfortable with a new way of being.

Another new mantra of mine is "Peace and flow feel like home." I get fidgety, and it feels boring, but the more I practice the life behaviors that bring peace and flow, the more comfortable my mind and body become. Every day that I act like a person who's mantra is "Peace and flow feel like home," by meditating, spending time in nature, practicing gratitude, being organized, I become that kind of person.

In James Clear's book *Atomic Habits*, he talks about making decisions based on the person you want to be. So, if I have decided to be a person who is peaceful and in flow, then every choice I make is either a vote for or against the person I want to be. The choices I make need to be the choices a peaceful person would make.

I wouldn't imagine the Dalai Lama rushing out of bed, downing two shots of espresso, and searching for his F*ing car keys!

My new management focuses on:
- Meditation
- Simplifying

What If It All Goes Right?

- Being in the moment
- Prayer
- Time in Nature
- Leaving and arriving everywhere early
- Getting plenty of rest
- Thinking well
- Eating well
- Limiting coffee
- Planning ahead
- Practicing mindfulness
- Getting and being organized
- Setting boundaries
- Saying yes to only the things I really want to do
- Saying no to the people, places, things, and events that make me feel stressed

To-Do List

Sometimes, the most important thing to add to your to do list is an apostrophe and two letters: So it goes from a "to-do list" to a "to-don't list."

I used to laugh when I would see someone with a to-do list of three things, but my list of fifty things never seemed to get done, so I have learned to simplify and cull it down to the essentials, and let the rest go!

In Practice

- If you have a suspicion that you might benefit from new management, take an inventory of the things that cause stress or any self-inflicted stress that can be eliminated.

- Create a new mantra for the way you live, and make daily choices that only that kind of person would make.

28. Fragile Faith

"All I have seen teaches me to trust the creator for all I have not seen."
—Ralph Waldo Emerson

It's been said, there are no atheists in foxholes. In the scariest moments—a flood, a hurricane, a diagnosis, a good-bye—being in a foxhole is a divine opportunity to ask ourself what we really believe.

I had my earliest religious experiences with a Methodist father and a recovering Baptist mother. My dad was a red-dirt Guthrie Oklahoma biscuits-and-gravy Methodist who held on to his religion, and my mother was a South Dakota recovering Baptist turned metaphysical.

We moved to California when I was four, and I just wanted a mother who wore pearls and baked bread and was still holding a hand duster when I walked in from school, as she floated in asking, "How was your day, dear?" But she came to age in the Mad-men days, wearing heels and making martinis, and she had reached ninja status for her typing and shorthand skills. She had been harassed and called broad, doll, and skirt, and by the time I came along, she was *over* it.

Scarlet Keys

So instead of June Cleaver from *Leave It to Beaver*, I got Shirley MacLaine. I had a mom who had a picture of Jesus on the wall but was reading tarot cards, holding crystals, and burning incense. I remember inviting a friend over, and when she said she had a headache, my mother offered to put her hands on her head and give her "energy." I would shrink with embarrassment until the next time that friend came over and said "Hey, can your mom do that thing on my head again?" The most popular boy in my high school once stopped by my house and asked if my mother was home so he could talk with her. She did have a magical way about her, and you could sit down in tears with her and hand her the pieces of your broken life, and she would just move them around like puzzle pieces and hand them back to you in a beautiful mosaic. When you walked away, everything was better.

But all of that interesting mix is a part of me. I like to very humbly use the word Christian when defining my beliefs and only in the sense of the radical mystic who preached love.

All religions are beautiful, and I believe all roads lead to the top of the mountain. So no religion is one-size-fits-all, and there are so many ways to believe. To me, God is too big to fit in one building, and we can't call him by the wrong name as long as we call him. Like when your grandmother's memory starts slipping, and she calls you by someone else's name, you don't mind because you know she loves you but isn't sure what to call you.

What If It All Goes Right?

I like the way going to church makes me feel, but I also find the divine in nature and in sunsets and in animals. In medicine, in music, in side-splitting laughter, and in other people.

Whatever it is we believe, or we don't believe, I'm convinced that something bigger than me designed the constellations and moonlight and me.

I don't know about you, but when things get so hard we don't think we can take another thing, it all comes down to either breathing or praying.

Here is my go-to prayer:

God, grant me the serenity
to accept the things I cannot change,
the courage to change the things I can,
and the wisdom to know the difference.
Amen

In Practice

- Where do you find something bigger than yourself?
- How can you strengthen your spiritual life?
- How can you take time each day to connect to the source that created you?
- The next time you are worried, hand it over to God, and then, turn your thoughts to something beautiful or fun or worthy of your attention.

29. Finding Fun

"We don't stop playing because we grow old; we grow old because we stop playing."

—George Bernard Shaw

When most teenagers grab the car keys to head out for the night, they often hear their mom or dad yell, "Be careful!" When I would walk out the door I would always hear my dad yell, "Have fun."

My dad was someone who understood the value of fun. When he was young, he remembered his father going to the bank to find out that the bank was closed and all of their money was gone. This was the great depression. So, he knew what hard times were, and after coming home after being in World War II as a soldier, he prized the rare and privileged act of having fun.

I can't remember ever going anywhere in the car with him when he wasn't singing, and he would always say things like, "When I travel for work, your mom thinks I'm out having a big time." And he was. He worked hard selling syndicated television shows and movies for Paramount Pictures, but he played well. He played golf, he swam, he watched great movies, he traveled, and he was funny and fun to be with. I was constantly caught off guard by the funny

What If It All Goes Right?

things he would say. My dad was a big guy, and one day I brought home cannoli cookies with powdered sugar and mini chocolate chips, and he said, "I need that like a snail needs air brakes." He made me laugh often, and we had a lot of fun together playing music, swimming, getting a Coke, and driving by the ocean.

Fun has gotten a bad rap in our productive to-do list society, along with other important restorative acts, like rest and napping. It feels frivolous. If we have fun, what would we have to show for it?

"Fun" and "play" often go hand in hand.

Playing like a kid can help adults live better lives. A 2013 Swiss study published in the *European Journal of Humor Research* showed that playful adults lived happier, more satisfying, healthier lives.

It turns out that having fun has its health benefits. When we have fun, according to a 2016 study done by scientists at Sahmyook University in Seoul, South Korea, the body releases the feel-good neurotransmitters dopamine and serotonin, which lead to elevated mood and a healthier cell-proliferation process.

For artists, when we take the time to have fun, we are more creative and work better after having fun. Think of Julia Cameron's books *The Artist's Way* and *The Artist's Date Book*.

Having fun with other people strengthens our relationships. I have seen that over and over again between my daughter and me. We have had a lot of fun together, and we always feel closer when we do.

Scarlet Keys

When I was a child, my friends and I knocked on each other's doors, and said, "Can you come out and play?" We wore glitter and ballet tutus to the grocery store. We were pirates and cowboys and mermaids. We played in dirt and made mud pies. We broke off branches for guns and put our wet hair up in a big towel so we could feel our long princess terrycloth hair. We had sticky faces and dirty feet and sang the songs to our favorite musicals at all times.

Later, fun turned into high school plays and cruising in our cars with the windows down and the radio up. We had long, stretched-out summer days, waves, and salted skin. Then college parties and concerts and finals and grades, graduation, and job hunting.

Then, fun became age-appropriate, more contained and buttoned up, as the bills stacked high and adulthood, jobs and parenthood were ushered in. But we get another chance to play when we have kids. We get a shower full of brightly colored squeaky toys and stuffed animals in our car. Dad accidentally goes to work with glitter in his beard and fabulously painted toenails, and Mom sits on floor playing Barbies. It's fun finding fun once again, with permission to be silly and light because it's important to make green eggs and ham and wear a sorting hat and drink butter beer at Harry Potter World and go to sleep with twinkly lights strewn across our ceiling.

As our children leave the nest and we pack up their toys and take down their posters from the wall, we need to save a little bit of that glitter for ourselves.

What If It All Goes Right?

As we find a new grey hair and blow out more candles on our cake, and as we change and get older, what we find fun, changes.

For me, now, fun is one more practice I have been pursing in the spirit of wellness. I am making fun a priority by taking Zumba classes, grabbing someone to play ping-pong with me, and trying new things.

I surveyed some dear friends of all ages, and here were the things my friends do for fun:

Phyllis G., Age 95
She writes for her local paper. She travels with her new husband Coni, whom she met on Match.com. She plays Mahjong. She walks her dog Lucky.

Patte B., Age 91
Maybe, because of my age, my fun is not too active. My most enjoyable time is spent cooking for company, chatting with friends (especially at lunch or dinner), playing Wordle and Connections, and discovering new places.

Betsy H., Age 87
Walking her little dog Loki, helping people in her community go to doctor's appointments, cooking, holding cocktail hour at her community home, playing poker.

Jack P., Age 81

Something I remember having, now replaced by smaller pleasures or more vital ones, like really enjoying a meal or having a meaningful talk with anybody, but especially close friends. Having gained knowledge into how the mind works, what really counts, attaining a deeper perception of reality and more wonderment at Life. These are gifts that this weird trip that I've been on has given me. It's not been fun, but it's provided me with deeper insight into my life.

Music has been and still remains a gift to mankind, a mirror of our emotions and Soul, and a terrific way to what would otherwise be inexpressible, and yes, it's fun.

Pat P., Ageless

Golf, writing poetry, reading poetry, riding a motorcycle, teaching, concerts.

Carole G., Age 70-something

My most fun is going to music: blues, mariachi, opera!!! We do that almost every night of the week and chat with musicians!

Larry Z., Ageless:

Likes to play piano, attend LIVE music—Jazz, Latin, Rock, and more, and go for long walks and take photographs!!! Also loves dining out and making new friends!!!

What If It All Goes Right?

Ariel H., Age 50
Being with my toddler. Enjoying meals out one on one with girlfriends to really talk and share deep connection and conversations. Bingeing TV series like The Bear.

In Practice

Finding Fun
- Make a list of things you used to do that are fun.
- When you make your to-do list, add something fun for the day.
- Make a list of things you've always wanted to try that are fun.
- Look at the local paper, and go see a show.
- Take a class to learn something new.
- Make a new friend.
- Try one new thing every month.
- When faced with a dreaded task, try to find a way to make it fun or more enjoyable: Playing fun music while doing taxes, eating ice-cream while doing the bills, listen to a standup comedian while driving in traffic.

30. Tigger and Eeyore

"Dismiss what insults your soul."
—Walt Whitman

Most of us don't have the luxury of sitting crossed legged on a mountain top with someone else washing our orange robe or our one rice bowl for us. Most of us have to navigate our emotional life down trafficked streets and moody teenagers and jobs, caring for an elderly parent or the everyday stress of looking for our F*ing keys.

Again, we will have difficult emotions—real things that need our attention, and we will have to feel them and learn what they have to teach us, because all a feeling wants is to be felt. But we can be selective and careful with the emotions we choose to nurture and steep ourselves in.

I've had to be vigilant about what I let in emotionally, because I've tuned into the concept of changing the environment of my body to afford the best chance to heal and be healthy. I have never been more aware of my internal life than when I was exhausted from chemotherapy. My world shrunk down to the emotional pinpoint of "tired." There was no room for anything else. I didn't have the luxury of low emotions, like resentments or worrying

What If It All Goes Right?

about something someone said, or spending time on a painful memory that bubbled up. Suddenly, these emotions were like a big, loud drunk stumbling in through the front door, and instead of making them tea, I began to usher them out.

Sometimes, we are going through chronic stress with things that are ongoing and have no known expiration date. But day to day, we can curate our thoughts and avoid toxic self-imposed emotions.

As I write this, I am awaiting test results. I found a small lump, and they took a biopsy, so in two or three days, I will know if I've had a recurrence or if it's just scar tissue. Now, this is when I get to practice the words I've written in this book. I have a weekend awaiting me, and I can either spend two days of my one precious life in complete terror with adrenaline and cortisol running through my body, or I can be in this one moment and live deep and wide.

Right now, I am writing this book, which is a total labor of love. I am sitting in my favorite cafe in a window seat with the afternoon sun warming me as trees release colored leaves that cartwheel in a windy flurry of red and yellow down red brick sidewalks. I'm sitting in front of a wall of cut flowers, and I will not let my imagination ruin a perfectly good day.

Whatever the news is, it can't steal this weekend. It can't have today.

I am steeped in gratitude and will spend the weekend in love, laughter, and joy.

It turns out that there is a hierarchy of emotions,

Scarlet Keys

and our bodies vibrate with higher or lower frequencies, depending on which ones we spend time in. Feeling good is a practice, and on a worst day, there are other emotions we can lean to.

When you think about the two characters from *Winnie the Pooh*, Tigger and Eeyore, what do you feel when you think of each one of them? Eeyore with his shoulders down, why-bother defeated voice, and Tigger bouncing through the world with a spring in his tail singing "The most wonderful thing about Tiggers is I'm the only one." Tigger is bright orange, and Eeyore is grey.

When you think of Eeyore you might associate him with emotions like depression and doubt and the color grey, and in this state, there may be emotions like:

boredom	*pessimism*	*frustration*
overwhelm	*disappointment*	*discouragement*
apathy	*worry*	*powerlessness*
unworthiness	*insecurity*	*blame*

And if Eeyore was to ever muster more energy to feel more intense emotions, he might lean into:

frustration	*impatience*	*irritation*	*anger*
revenge	*hatred*	*rage*	*jealousy*
fear	*grief*	*depression*	*powerlessness*
victim	*repair*	*guilt*	*shame*

What If It All Goes Right?

In the land of Tigger, you might assign emotions like enthusiasm, joy, and optimism, and the color orange, and the following list:

trust *knowledge* *love*

appreciation *passion* *hopefulness*

eagerness *contentment* *positive expectation*

belief

If Tigger were to ever win the lottery or go sky diving, he might move into:

bliss *euphoria* *elation*

exuberancy *exhilaration* *ebulliency*

When we are guarding our hearts, it's important to notice the quality of emotions that different people, places, and activities evoke in us. Some people thrive on gossiping or a slow-death-by-small-talk, and I start looking for exit signs. I walk away feeling drained and sometimes overwhelmed. The same thing with activities, noticing how we feel after an encounter. Does that person or event leave me drained, triggered, or exhausted, or do we feel lighter and happier?

By the way, the tests I had been waiting for came back negative. I'm so glad I didn't waste my time imagining the worst.

In Practice

- Who are the Tiggers in your life? The cheerleaders? The people who make you laugh and inspire you?
- Who are the energy vampires, and how can you set boundaries around them?
- What are activities that make you feel alive and give you energy?
- What are the activities or places that leave you feeling drained or heavy?
- Make a habit of spending time with Tiggers and doing things that give you energy.
- Make a list of people places and things that leave you in a higher vibrational state.
- Practice these high vibration states.
- Meditate and think back to vacations, events, people, and places that elicit these high-vibration feeling states, and put your hand over your heart. Bring up that feeling, maybe close your eyes, and try adding a smile.
- Remember a moment of love, recall how that felt, and access that feeling as often as you can.

31. The Hardest Thing

"You must do the thing you think you cannot do."
—Eleanor Roosevelt

We all have a warrior inside of us. We are made for hard things. We might not know it yet, but we always rise to the occasion.

One in eight woman are diagnosed with breast cancer.

I had found a lump in my left breast, and now, I was sitting on a cold table on my birthday, in a gown, staring eye-to-eye with my radiologist, trying to say the "C" word. I couldn't even say it. All I could manage was, "Do I have…," and she responded, "Are you asking me?" and I said, "I guess I am," and she said, "Yes, you have two tumors and invasive ductal carcinoma."

My heart fell like an elevator down a hundred floors with no cable. I was unable to speak.

After the biopsy results were returned, I found out that I had an aggressive form of breast cancer but that it was treatable. Now, the wimpiest person in the world—afraid to take a single Tylenol—was facing chemotherapy, a double mastectomy, and immunotherapy drugs.

Scarlet Keys

In a flurry of weeks, I had to find an oncologist and a surgeon. I also had to decide if I wanted to enter a trial or do traditional therapy, and then figure out how to tell my fourteen-year-old daughter that her mother had cancer. I held that news inside my heart like water breaking through cracks in a dam for a week before I had all of the information and a treatment plan.

When I sat her down to tell her, through our flood of tears, I said, "We can do this. We can do hard things, and this is our plan. And soon, you will have the best hair and boobs in this house." I can't believe I managed to get a slight smile to curve on her little lips. I knew she would follow my emotional lead and that my attitude would steer her experience.

I was scared and overwhelmed, but I had a moment of clarity when I thought, "How do I want to be as I go through all of this?" I knew it was going to be hard and scary. But I also knew that there were other things it could be. So I decided to walk through it with grace.

I realized I wasn't unarmed. I wasn't an untrained warrior thrown on to the battlefield. I was a woman who was about to find out that every moment of her life had trained her for the hardest thing.

Three people recommended the book *Preparing for Surgery*, by Peggy Huddleston. Huddleston mentions that we are in a suggestive state in the moments right before we are going under anesthesia and as we are coming out. She suggests that we write out a list of affirmations to be read by the anesthesiologist just as

What If It All Goes Right?

we are going under and just as we are waking up. We can print it out and tape it to our chest for them to read.

Huddleston has a meditation to do for a week or two before surgery: to visualize the best outcome. The best outcome, hmmm…. Could I push through the fog of dread and expect the best? She suggested calling the anesthesiologist and talking with her beforehand.

So I called my anesthesiologist and asked if she would read my affirmations. She said she'd read anything I gave her. I asked, "Even a rap?" and she said "Even a rap." It is a well-known fact that laughter is medicine, and I was determined to pick it up and carry it into battle with me.

Being a musician and songwriter, I carefully curated a listening playlist to be played during my surgery, and my surgeon agreed to play it. I wrote my surgeon a rap, of course, setting the tone for any levity I could muster. I mean how many songwriting professors does she operate on? She loved it and said it actually gave her teenagers a reason to think she was cool, "'cuz now it's Dr. Molly Buzdon in da house."

In the days and weeks preceding my surgery, my brain went into Fear Mode and worst-case scenarios. I know our prehistoric brains haven't evolved far from a state of constant vigilance against saber-toothed tigers, and we have a negativity bias. But imagining the worst is a false sense of control, similar to how rehearsing tragedy somehow makes it easier or can prepare us. But it's just imagination. I realized that I didn't want to do that to myself, and my cortisol wasn't helping the matter, so if the worst outcome is only my imagination, why not imagine the best outcome? Dare I hope? Dare I ask the question, what if it all goes right? What if this team of doctors are wonderful? What if I can look for the best? What if something good can be found along the way?

The day of my surgery, I brought a wireless speaker in the room and did my meditation. While sitting there in my robe, waiting to be taken in, I asked my husband if he would dance for me. I know it's ridiculous, but laughter is healing, and transformative, so I searched Spotify's playlists and accidentally clicked on "Stripper Tunes."

The poor guy, trying to dance to Cardi B in a hospital waiting room. But he did it, and he brought it. It was a bit like Will Ferrell lap dancing. He grabbed a chair, sat in it backwards like Jennifer Beals in *Flashdance*, and then turned the chair around, arched his back, and kicked his legs into the air with his Boy Scout, Catholic, kind, and scared face, trying to make his terrified wife laugh. He did. I am sure the nurses outside the door were wondering what was going on, but I didn't care because I was laughing so hard that my anxiety couldn't catch its breath. That deep laughter ushered the fear and the worry out of the room.

After my surgery, I woke up feeling rested and clear-headed. It was during COVID, when visitor access was restricted, but my dear friend who is a

What If It All Goes Right?

midwife at the hospital was able to hang out with me for four hours in my room. There was an extra IV poll that wasn't being used, and she dared me to do a pole dance to send to my husband since I owed him one. I did it to the tune of "What a Feeling" from *Flashdance*, but it was more like Betty White than Jennifer Beals. I was reveling in relief, and we laughed so hard. Once again, anxiety was asked to leave the room. It had all gone right.

There was so much more ahead. I had twelve rounds of chemo to face. Each week, I walked into the infusion center as a different version of myself depending on how I was feeling. The first week, I was so scared that I walked in small and quiet in one long constant prayer of "I am surrounded by white light, and bless this day, and thank you for healing me, and I am safe." I had made a flower arrangement from my garden to give to the nurses as a thank you. Week 2, I felt fragile but needed to feel brave, so I wore my Superman T-shirt. Then week 3, I remember parking the car, and I felt like I was walking through smoke in all black leather like a superhero with a heavy metal soundtrack.

Week after week, I would find a new avatar, from Gandhi to Superwoman. I remember, about week 9, I walked in singing, "I'm fucking here, I'm fucking here, let's just get this shit over with!" Some days, I walked in, filled with gratitude and maybe even laughing. Because, yes, it was hard, but it was also other things, and I got to decided what else it could be.

Scarlet Keys

It's a lot to ask of a partner, to lean on them emotionally for everything, or to take time off work to take you to every appointment. My husband Greg was holding up our entire world, working full time, walking the dog, helping with housework, being King of the Laundry, and then trying to make me laugh on the impossible days. Words can never express my gratitude for my amazing husband. Also, I didn't want to overburden him.

When people say, "Let me know if you ever need a ride, or anything at all," we just never ask, because we don't want to burden them. So, to have my dear friend Susan say "I'm taking you to your appointments" was such a gift to give me and my family. We don't realize how we can help a family when we help share the burden of care. Community is vital, but having true friends is everything.

Susan would drive all the way from Boston to New Hampshire, and then we'd drive to Maine for treatment. Some days, we would laugh, some days I would cry and walk arm-in-arm with her into the treatment center. Most days, we'd drive to the ocean, and I'd take my shoes off and put my feet in the cold water to ward off neuropathy, and do my earthing, and be with nature, and then we'd go to lunch.

Many days, I would say, "I had so much fun with you today. Oh wait, I had chemo."

A good friend is a balm to your soul, and that kind of support is priceless. She did so many little thoughtful things, like buying me a long thin pillow to protect my chest when I drove with the seat

What If It All Goes Right?

belt on, to starting a GoFundMe page to help with things that weren't covered by insurance. She did the greatest thing any friend could do, which is to spend time with me and just be my friend.

There were so many silver linings on my cloudiest of days. If we have just one true friend in this world, we are lucky.

After my chemo was finished, I had a year of an infusion drug to directly treat my form of cancer. On my last day of treatment, I had gone to the bathroom, and when I returned to my room, Susan had decorated it. Across my chair was a sign that read "Celebrate."

After the final treatment was complete, I got in the car and turned to Susan, bursting into tears, as I said, "I can't believe I just did all that."

No one is ever out of the woods. We live in the woods, and we never know what will happen next or when we will take our last breath. But we get to decide how we will walk through this crazy, amazing, unpredictable life.

I hope that when you walk through your hardest thing, with your fear and dread, that you also bring your grace, gratitude, joy, loved ones, and even laughter, because we get to bring it all with us.

In Practice

- Practice reaching for emotions that raise your vibration to a higher feeling state.
- Try imagining the best outcome for anything you're worried about.
- When you veer off to a fear-based thought, practice shifting your thoughts back to the best possible outcome.
- Practice feeling the way you would feel if you knew everything was going to go well.

Afterword

Thank you for joining me—and especially, if it was your own hardest thing that brought you here. Now, together, we go forward. I hope that you find comfort and strength in what I am sharing here. So, let's get to nap bragging and making down time. Remember that making your family a quiche or sitting with a good friend over coffee is the true accomplishment.

Please make living well your priority. Practice wielding the word "no" with wild abandon. Become a guilt-free boundary boss.

Let's start a revolution of doing less—even doing nothing. Remember that we are human *be*-ings. All you need to do is be.

I hope that this book found you on a day when you needed it. That something in here has turned up the light on your day, a bit, and reminded you that you are not alone.

You've got this. Whatever "this" is, you've got it! You were made for hard things, and You. Have. Got. This!

Life will always challenge us. That's just part of the deal. But as my father Charlie Keys used to say, "If it wasn't this, it'd be something else, so you might as well enjoy yourself."

Be well.

Scarlet Keys

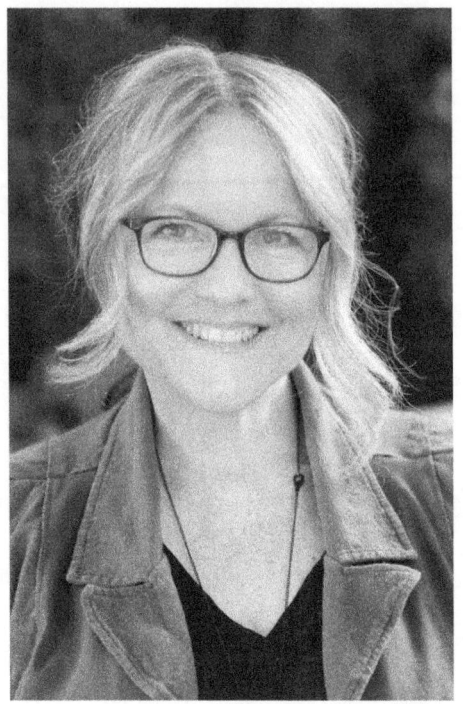

Photo by Mim Adkins

Scarlet Keys is a professor at Berklee College of Music, an award-winning songwriter, host of the podcast *What's in a Song*, author of the book *The Craft of Songwriting*, and an inspirational speaker.

Some of her past students include Laufey, Lizzy McAlpine, Charlie Puth, and Amy Allen.

She lives in New Hampshire with her husband, daughter, their dog Sunny, and the world's sweetest rescue cats.

Printed in the USA
CPSIA information can be obtained
at www.ICGtesting.com
JSHW020315280424
61851JS00002B/6

9 798218 339883